"Signe Darpinian has given us a much-needed guide to navigating menopause without shame or diet culture. With warmth, wisdom, and evidence-based insight, this book helps women understand their changing bodies and emotions while building a more peaceful relationship with food and self. A must-read for anyone ready to embrace midlife with compassion and confidence."

Jenn Salib Huber, RD, ND, CIEC, *host of* The Midlife Feast *podcast and author of* Eat To Thrive During Menopause: Managing Your Symptoms with Nourishing Foods

"We can finally exhale! As a registered dietitian and eating disorder specialist, I am thrilled to find a menopause guide that I can recommend without the diet and fitness hype and the scales and belly-blasting looming in the center! How refreshing to find solid advice for navigating menopause that encourages self-trust and drops the body shaming and fear-mongering."

Deb Benfield, MEd, RDN/LDN, RYT, *author of* Unapologetic Aging: How to Mend and Nourish Your Relationship with Your Body

"As a menopause physician, my patients are always asking for resources to help them through this hormonal transition and all of the changes their bodies are experiencing. There is so much noise out there on social media and beyond promoting unsafe practices and I am grateful for Signe's book detailing evidence based approaches to health! This book is now part of the 'menopause library' I recommend for my patients!"

Amy J Voedisch, MD, MS, MSCP, *author of* Estrogen, Interrupted: A Guide to Surviving and Thriving in Perimenopause

"This book offers a thoughtful and supportive approach to navigating menopause without focusing on weight as a measure of health or worth. The author, Signe Darpinian – a therapist with experience in the weight inclusive space, provides practical guidance and compassionate insight to help readers feel more at home in their bodies during this transition. It's a reassuring resource for anyone looking for an alternative to the usual weight-centered messages around menopause."

Naomi Busch MD, MSCP, *owner of Seattle Menopause Medicine*

"How I wish Signe's book had been available as I made my journey through menopause! This book's combination of factual medical information, enlightening personal stories, and non-judgmental, wise, and gentle guidance makes it a must-read for all who wish to go through menopause in community rather than isolation. Menopause is a natural process, and Signe helps her readers find kindness for their changing bodies."

Connie Sobczak, *co-founder of The Body Positive and author of* Embody: Learning to Love Your Unique Body (and quiet that critical voice!)

"Have you ever opened a book and felt as if every word was written directly to and for you? Signe Darpinian's warm, compassionate, and candid book demystifies a phase of life few of us were ever taught about, standing in as a (highly knowledgeable) older sister who wants only to help readers – her collective 'little sisters' – flourish in midlife and beyond. This book found me at the right moment in time – Ophelia is alive and well and experiencing hot flashes! – and I can't wait to witness its impact on a generation of women. Culturally, individually, we NEED this book!"

Sara Pipher Gilliam, *co-author*, Reviving Ophelia 25th Anniversary Edition

"The time for menopause being a shameful problem for individual women to try and navigate, fix, or hide away on their own, instead of a universal experience deserving attention and care, is over. With books like this, there is no longer any need to feel shame, diet, or think there is something wrong with your body, or you. *You and your body are not the problem*. The problem has been lack of education, research, treatment, and community for women experiencing menopause. (Also, if you are grieving, the symptoms peri/menopause and grief are shockingly similar. You're not going crazy. You're grieving, and in peri/menopause.) Thank God/dess, and Signe, that problem is now being addressed in this book!"

Linda Shanti McCabe, PsyD, *author of* The Recovery Mama's Guide to your Eating Disorder Recovery in Pregnancy and Postpartum *and* After Your Person Dies

"As more and more wellness influencers promote risky 'solutions' for the symptoms of the menopause transition, it's harder than ever for midlife women to find guidance they can trust. Thank goodness for Darpinian's book, which provides empathetic, evidence-based guidance for women to take care of their physical and emotional well-being during this phase of life. No gimmicks, no fad diets, just expert advice shared with wit and wisdom."

Oona Hanson, *parent educator*

"Finally – a menopause guide that ditches the diets, quick fixes, and shame. As an eating disorder specialist, I'm grateful for this weight-inclusive, compassionate resource that helps women navigate midlife with self-acceptance and tools to manage changing bodies, sleep, emotions, and more!"

Wendy Sterling, MS, RD, CSSD, CEDS-C, *author of* How to Nourish Yourself Through an Eating Disorder: Recovery for Adults with the Plate-by-Plate Approach®

"Understanding menopause is crucial for providing effective and empathetic care, either as a treatment provider or as a friend or partner. *A Woman's Guide to Menopause, Body Image, and Emotional Well-being at Midlife* skillfully addresses the physical and emotional changes women experience during this transition – knowledge and attunement that are foundational to cultivating stronger relationships, resulting in better therapeutic outcomes."

Riley Nickols, PhD, CEDS-C, *counseling and sport psychologist, founder of Mind Body Endurance LLC*

"Perimenopause can be such a confusing time for many women, and with the lack of research, as well as the overabundance of information, it can make it very challenging to know the right path to take in helping to mitigate one's symptoms. Signe's book, *A Women's Guide to Menopause, Body Image and Emotional Well-being at Midlife* is a true godsend. Very rarely can you find information discussing this transformative period without the discussion of GLP-1s for intentional weight loss, or the need to do intermittant fasting, which is not necessarily appropriate for everyone. Signe, with her background and experience writing about eating disorders and disordered eating, turns that same lens onto this period of one's life and looks at helping us understand why the change in hormones causes an increase in adiposity or more joint pain thus limiting movement. Looking at how we can eat, move and bring in more positive and healthy relationships are all important tenets in this book and can help build a strong foundation as we enter this new stage of life. This book helps to solidify that this does not have to be a scary and anxiety-provoking time but one of growth, transformation and knowing that you are not alone on this journey."

Anietie Ukpe-Wallace, PT, DPT, *author of* Tending to Your Womb: A Journey of Joy, Grief and Self-Discovery

A Woman's Guide to Menopause, Body Image, and Emotional Well-being at Midlife

A Woman's Guide to Menopause, Body Image, and Emotional Well-being at Midlife is the definitive primer for all things midlife and menopause, offering anticipatory guidance and research-based strategies.

This book breaks down the transition to menopause in an accessible way to guide readers through what can be a confusing and isolating life stage. Harnessing her trademark curiosity and relatable wit, Signe Darpinian helps women navigate the most common menopause symptoms, body changes, and mental health and emotional challenges, and tackles love, sex, and body image through a weight-inclusive lens. Each chapter shares real life stories and expert advice to empower women to cut through diet-culture's harmful messaging and foster their own authentic well-being and joy.

Ideal for women approaching or experiencing menopause or as a clinical companion for those working with this population, this guide is essential for traversing menopause and midlife.

Signe Darpinian, LMFT, CEDS, is a public speaker and therapist who specializes in eating disorders and body image across the lifespan. Her books include *No Weigh!* and *Raising Body Positive Teens*. She is the creator and host of the personal growth podcast *Therapy Rocks!*

SIGNE DARPINIAN

A Woman's Guide

to Menopause, Body Image, and Emotional Well-being at Midlife

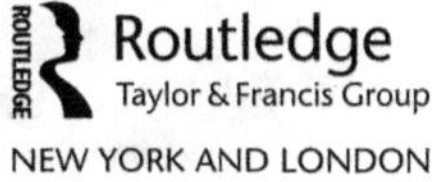

NEW YORK AND LONDON

Designed cover image: Getty Images

First published 2026
by Routledge
605 Third Avenue, New York, NY 10158

and by Routledge
4 Park Square, Milton Park, Abingdon, Oxon, OX14 4RN

Routledge is an imprint of the Taylor & Francis Group, an informa business

ISBN: 9781041053156 (hbk)
ISBN: 9781041053187 (pbk)
ISBN: 9781003632245 (ebk)

DOI: 10.4324/9781003632245

Typeset in Joanna
by Deanta Global Publishing Services, Chennai, India

This book is for Andie – the love of my life, who inspires everything I do – and for generations of women to come. May you have the resources and the wisdom you need to traverse menopause with ease and grace.

Contents

Acknowledgments

Mom, you were right about everything, especially my hormones! Thank you for knowing me better than anyone and telling me I needed hormones even when my doctor didn't.

To my daughter, Andie, for reminding me of our family motto, "you won't get a yes unless you ask," while I was pitching this book idea, and for your GIFs that got me to the finish line ("You are amazing, you've got this, your book is going to be awesome!") I love you more than anything in the entire universe. I'm sorry you had to wear dirty socks that time, and for all the cereal dinners – please don't unlearn how to do the laundry.

I owe so much to every expert that said yes to me when I asked them for contributions from their areas of expertise. This book wouldn't be the same without each of you. Dr. Amy Voedisch deserves special mention – thank you for co-writing Chapter One and bringing in your contraception and menopause expertise to the book; Dr. Naomi Busch for the most awesome vignettes in Chapters One and Two, and for taking the time to give me guidance when I needed it. You went above and beyond for me; Dr. Abby Cobb-Walch for your excerpt on transgender and gender diverse menopause considerations; Julie Dillon Duffy for your contribution on PCOS in midlife in the middle of your own book launch; Val Schonberg, for being my first teacher in the menopause space, and for the "Is it Perimenopause or is it REDs" section.

Dr. Riley Nickols, thank you for your REDs section, marriage analogy in the body image chapter, and continued moral support; Dr. Cynthia Bulik thank you for advising me through the genetics of eating disorders section and steering me in the right direction in the disordered eating chapter; Dr. Jennifer Gaudiani for the most badass weight-inclusive vignette I could have ever dreamed of; Dr. Anietie Ukpe-Wallace, you taught me so much about the importance of pelvic health in midlife and beyond; Dr. Kelly McGonigal for the research on how movement makes us happy; Dr. Joanna Steinglass for the neuroscience of habit section; Jenn Salib Huber, your "gentle nutrition" section is perfection; Brenna O'Malley, thank you for the tips on managing body image distress when looking at photographs of ourselves; Crystal Johnson for the wisdom you bring to group fitness, the absence of diet-culture in class, and for making strength training fun!

To my therapist friends and colleagues: Dr. Linda Shanti, thank you for improving my grief literacy, and sharing your midlife widowhood journey with us; Margaret Hunter, I cried so hard when I read the beautiful story of your mother, and the art therapy process at the end; Dr. Brenda Schaeffer, your entire section on "midlife relationship themes" is a master class; Dr. Ashley Brauer, you gave me so much of your time and expertise on sleep and I learned so much from you; Suzannah Neufeld for helping me adapt my favorite skill from your book to the menopause transition; and Dr. Elizabeth Laugeson, thank you for taking the time to let me interview you and ask *all* the friendship questions!

I want to acknowledge all of the individuals who shared their personal stories in this book. You took the time to share stories that will make a difference in the lives of others. These stories are the heart of the book. Nik, thank you for sharing your transgender perspective, I feel so happy knowing that you are happy; Connie Sobczak for "the art of aging," section, climbing, and reclaiming "old age"; Virgie Tovar for normalizing bloody sheets and body positivity as a relationship value; Catherine, your empty nest story made me bawl like a baby, thank you; Luciana Naldi for showing us how to strive for a new definition of beauty after hair loss; Helen for giving me your blessing to share your life's journey with food and body image; to Jessie for shining a light on "symbolic losses" such as body image grief; Maeve for "Bringing Sexy Back," and giving us a template for taking valued action; Alexsia thank you for your authentic story about your journey through insomnia, it will help so many people who are suffering in silence; Elia thank you for reminding us of the joys of having movement in our lives, and sharing it with friends; Luzi I adore your humor and laughs about your real life urban farm, and an occasional rat; Rachel for increasing our awareness about brain fog and sharing your struggle; and Victoria for sharing your life journey with us as a stunning coda for this book.

Thank you to my midlife female friends that endured the last couple of years hearing about this project; Stephanie, Jenny, Tracy, Jen, Alexa, Runa. Forgive me for my hypervigilance about your possible menopause symptoms; "Did you skip a period? Or two?", "Have you had a hot flash?", "Are you anxious?", "Did you get weepy?", "How's your sleep?", "A UTI?!", "Do you need a pad?", "A pill?", "OMG, it's vaginal atrophy!!!"

To Holly Marian Davies who gave me this book idea to begin with, and said I could do it, even when I didn't think I could. Thank you for teaching me about all of the beautiful rainbows in the world, you are my rainbow.

Thank you to Dr. Shelley Aggarwal and Wendy Sterling, my co-authors from *No Weigh!* and *Raising Body Positive Teens*. They say having co-authors is like a marriage – I married very, very well. I love and appreciate you both. I'm so grateful for the time you both took to help me with so many aspects of this book. You were both there for me when I needed you – flashback to when I texted you about one book section, "I'm too dumb to dumb this down!" I won't ever forget your friendship and support.

Thank you to Sophie Dracott and Amanda Savage at Routledge: Taylor & Francis Group, for "getting" my vision for a crossover book, and allowing me to write it in a way that's in alignment with me…and for all the laughs along the way.

A most special thanks to Sara Pipher for spinning my straw into gold and taking me to the finish line. I trust you and your judgement immensely. You are my ride or die. I could not have done this without you.

Author's Note

Traditionally, women's health and well-being have not been a health-care or medical research priority. Unfortunately, this has fundamentally affected health equity and outcomes for women (Balch, 2024). Further, I recognize that those assigned female at birth will go through menopause, but not everyone who experiences menopause identifies as female. More research and consideration are needed about menopause in transgender men and gender-diverse people. In this book, I focus primarily on women experiencing midlife and menopause, but I hope that it is a helpful resource for all who choose to read it. Additional resources are cited in the resource section at the back of the book.

REFERENCE

Balch, B. (2024, March 26). *Why we know so little about women's health*. AAMC. Retrieved May 21, 2025, from https://www.aamc.org/news/why-we-know-so-little-about-women-s-health

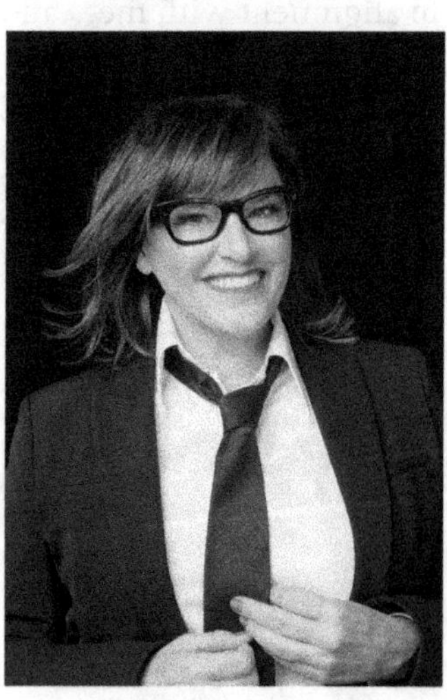

Credit: Photograph by Jenny Elia Pfeiffer

Preface

My path to the patch – the *estrogen patch*, that is – was like Tim Burton's titular *Alice in Wonderland* trying to find her way out of the Queen of Hearts' garden maze. It started with bouts of insomnia, hot flashes, urinary incontinence, and joint pain that sporadically made it intolerable to be in a sitting position and uncomfortable to walk, especially in the morning. This was complemented by hair loss and seemingly whimsical body changes, including a new layer of midsection adiposity, and a dramatic increase in breast size that startled even my own mother!

For me the changes weren't just physical. I began experiencing waves of anxiety and depression, something I hadn't grappled with before. Panic attacks became so unpredictable that I never knew if one might hit me while I was driving my car. I was intentional about the music I played while driving, a tool I prescribe often to my own clients, because music has the ability to pull us out of our current emotional state. I used other Dialectical Behavioral Therapy (DBT) skills I dole out daily like "Cope Ahead" before getting in the car, and imagining "how good it could possibly go." Nothing helped. I started to wonder if I could only socialize if I got rides with other people. I was embarrassed to tell anyone that it felt debilitating to drive.

Crying randomly became a regular occurrence. This even happened when I was happy. For example, I saw a post about Freddie Mercury being known to carry around a birthday book so he'd never forget a friend's birthday. Bawled like a baby. This phenomenon is anecdotally called "crying over dog food commercials."

Of course, I also cried when I was sad. The last time that happened, I tried so hard to hold the tears back in front of my daughter that the buildup became too big and the dam broke. She put her hand on mine and said, "It's going to be okay Mom, would you like me to make you some green tea?"

In my whimpering, crackling voice, tears running down my face, I sniffled, "I don't like tea." Oh great! I was inviting my child in to regulate my emotions. I know better than this, I'm a therapist!

I remember saying to my OB/GYN, "I don't know what's happening to me, and the only way I can describe it to you is that it feels like I have arthritis all over my body." I left the office with a referral to physical therapy, where my forearm was massaged with a scraping tool for one hour (to be fair I also had tennis elbow for the first time in my tennis life). Soon after, I received a $900 bill, which of course made me cry, because everything did.

I don't like to mistake a Google search for a medical degree, but I finally did one because I thought I was going crazy. I typed, "Why would a 51-year-old woman be experiencing joint pain?" The answer was immediate: "As estrogen levels decline during perimenopause (the first stage of menopause), the joints can swell and become painful."

I would discover much later in my menopause studies that 50 percent of women have joint pain at menopause. It's called "arthralgia" (Panay et al., 2024). How could I not have known this was coming? Why didn't my doctor mention this? Maybe she was going to discuss hormone therapy (HT) if the physical therapy didn't resolve my joint pain. Or…is it possible my doctor did not have menopause knowledge? As it turns out, fewer than one in five gynecologists receive formal training in menopause (Krewson, 2023). A "heads-up" that 51 is the most common age for menopause onset would have been amazing (Aljumah et al., 2023). It's not as if we don't have existing templates for how bodies change; think Sex Ed before puberty hits. "Hey, your voice might sound a little like a harmonica in the near future, and that's okay," or "You might expect some armpit hair and acne soon, also natural."

But, "The increase in adipose tissue, especially for biological females? Yep, it's on its way to protect your fertility organs." Rarely spoken. Imagine if it was the norm to start similar discussions with women in their mid-thirties, in order to prepare them for the menopause transition (Santoro, 2024). "You might see an increase in adiposity around your midsection due to depleted estrogen. The body is physiologically trying to help us out, this time by producing a different type of estrogen through our fat cells. Hot flashes, night sweats, and sleep disturbances: This is all a natural part of the process." This way women could use the knowledge to set up support for themselves if needed, rather than judging themselves for feeling confused.

If your menopause story is anything like mine, you probably won't be surprised to learn that women are rarely referred to a menopause specialist by their OB/GYN (Wolf, 2018). By the time I self-referred to a specialist at a hormone clinic, I was in bad shape mentally and physically, and desperate to figure out how to ameliorate my menopausal symptoms. Alas, the hormone clinic was understaffed and I waited two months for an appointment.

Once I finally met with my specialized care team to determine the best path for my treatment, based on the benefits and risks I presented with, I was prescribed a twice-weekly estrogen patch (applied transdermally) along with nightly oral progesterone. This combination is called estrogen plus progesterone therapy (EPT). I look back at my journal during those days, and I had scrawled countless illegible entries just trying to journal my way through the distress. I passed endless days waiting for my insurance company to approve my particular hormone therapy combination. I spent hours on the phone, each time dealing with a new person on the other end, intermittent rudeness, and occasionally being hung up on or yelled at. When the prescription finally came through I was unspeakably relieved. This had been a spiritual practice for sure.

It took a week for the added hormones to stabilize my symptoms, and for me it was magical. My joint pain started to relent, my mood stabilized, and my hot flashes and night sweats disappeared. Confession: Before the HT kicked in, I was secretly awaiting my follow up appointment so I could finally tell my doctor at the hormone clinic how awfully I had been treated. But by the time my appointment arrived, I was in such a balanced place that I couldn't muster any complaints. When the doctor asked, "How is it going?" I extolled, "Great, it's amazing, thank you. It's working so well I want more!" (She said no.)

I imagine that if my menopause transition was a smooth one, I wouldn't feel compelled to write a book on the topic. But here we are! As a therapist who specializes in eating disorders and body image, I struggled to find books and resources that aligned with my values of living and practicing from a non-diet approach. Many of the existing menopause books focus on changing your body, dieting, and exercising in a way that is not sustainable. While we know that some weight gain and redistribution is common during menopause, the reasons why are complex, and have to do with hormonal fluctuation and aging. Regardless of the reasons, dieting is largely unsuccessful (Wolf, 2018) (Sumithran et al., 2011), and studies show that the cycle of losing weight then re-gaining weight (called "weight cycling") has negative impacts on health (Swartz et al., 2025). I wanted to offer a guide to learn about what's happening in your body without selling a narrative that your body is wrong and needs to change. Therefore, the content you'll find here stems from a weight-inclusive lens, because the last thing we need is *more* diet culture in the menopause space.

Menopause is a highly personal experience; not everyone's menopause transition will be highly symptomatic like mine. A proportion of women will go through menopause with few or no symptoms and as such will not require treatment. Some women might choose HT but have a longer trial and error period than I did. And some will be symptomatic, but not able to take hormones due to their medical history and risk factors. Others will find that hormones just aren't the right path for them. Ultimately, we don't want to treat menopause as a medical condition – it's a natural part of aging – nor do we want to trivialize distressing symptoms. There are many ways to manage menopause symptoms, and they are not all hormone based. No matter where you are on your journey, this book will provide a roadmap to help you navigate your transition with as much ease as possible.

In the pages to follow, you'll find that each chapter shares stories from individuals with a range of different experiences, in hopes that you will see yourself reflected and know that you are not alone. I've also included skills and tools in each chapter; the bigger the offering of interventions, the easier it will be to pick and choose what is right for you. Interactive prompts will help you integrate the material as well as reduce emotionally aroused states. If you keep practicing them, you will get really good at knowing what skills you should use based on the current emotional state you're in, whether that challenge is related to fluctuating hormones and mood, body image concerns, interpersonal effectiveness, sleep, or eating difficulties.

Part One of this book includes the basics of menopause, your changing body, and the most common symptoms and treatments to date. Part Two focuses on understanding your changing emotions and cultivating mental health by bringing awareness to common midlife themes and offering tools to help you navigate challenges skillfully. It's also about providing protective factors for disordered eating and eating disorders, which are on the rise in this life phase. Part Three discusses embodying a diet-free lifestyle and understanding alternatives to fad diets. This includes learning how to eat in response to your body's wisdom, building body image resilience, and moving in ways that feel sustainable to you. Finally, Part Four focuses on enhancing midlife through friendship, romantic relationships, and sexual health.

I'm happy to report that, as of this writing, my daughter no longer has to offer me tea, and I can *mostly* drive with ease. I am thoroughly enjoying the wisdom and self awareness that comes from being in midlife. I have gratitude for my exact experience through the menopause transition; without it I wouldn't have the understanding and compassion I do, coupled with a deep desire to help other women feel less isolated through their own experiences. My hope is that the skills and tools in this guide will lay the foundation for you to be able to embrace your own midlife journey. I look forward to the evolution of our menopause awareness, discussion, knowledge, and treatment.

Remember, after a series of strange events, Alice did make it through Wonderland and back into her own reality. She was changed by her experiences for the better. Whether it's patches or pills, yoga or joyful new friendships – or some combination of all these and more – we will get through this together.

REFERENCES

Aljumah, R., Phillips, S., & Harper, J. C. (2023). An online survey of postmenopausal women to determine their attitudes and knowledge of the menopause. *Post Reproductive Health*, 29(2), 67–84. https://doi.org/10.1177/20533691231166543

Krewson, C. (2023, August 11). *Survey shows menopause curriculums lacking in residency programs*. Contemporary OB/GYN. https://www.contemporaryobgyn.net/view/survey-shows-menopause-curriculums-lacking-in-residency-programs

Panay, N., Ang, S. B., Cheshire, R., Goldstein, S. R., Maki, P., Nappi, R. E., & on behalf of the International Menopause Society Board. (2024). Menopause and mht in 2024: Addressing the key controversies – an international menopause society white paper. *Climacteric*, 27(5), 441–457. https://doi.org/10.1080/13697137.2024.2394950

Santoro, N. (2024). Basics of the menopause transition. *Menopause*, 31(10), 921–922. https://doi.org/10.1097/GME.0000000000002423

Sumithran, P., Prendergast, L. A., Delbridge, E., Purcell, K., Shulkes, A., Kriketos, A., & Proietto, J. (2011). Long-term persistence of hormonal adaptations to weight loss. *New England Journal of Medicine*, 365(17), 1597–1604. https://doi.org/10.1056/NEJMoa1105816

Swartz, A. Z., Wood, K., Farber-Eger, E., Petty, A., & Silver, H. J. (2025). Weight trajectory impacts risk for 10 distinct cardiometabolic diseases. *The Journal of Clinical Endocrinology & Metabolism*, dgaf348. https://doi.org/10.1210/clinem/dgaf348

Wolf, J. (2018, July 20). *Doctors don't know how to treat menopause symptoms*. AARP. https://www.aarp.org/health/conditions-treatments/menopause-symptoms-doctors-relief-treatment/

PART 1
Your Changing Body

What Is Menopause, Really?

One

Co-written by Amy J Voedisch, MD, MS, MSCP

When Sarah was 44 years old, she started to experience sudden changes in her mood. She noticed that the littlest things irritated her and she found herself feeling impatient with her children and husband. At work, she occasionally became weepy and felt a general sense of overwhelm. One night, she woke at 2 a.m. and discovered her sheets were drenched with sweat. It dawned on her that she might be entering perimenopause.

Sarah began to read and listen to everything she could. Her social media was flooded with perimenopause and menopause influencers telling her that she should see her doctor and discuss her symptoms. She scheduled an appointment with her primary care physician (PCP) and was surprised to find out that her doctor did not feel that they could treat her. They explained they did not learn about menopause in medical school and referred her to a gynecologist.

After waiting several weeks (some people wait months) to be seen, Sarah was hopeful that she would finally get some help. She explained to the gynecologist that she'd never had mood symptoms before and didn't have a history of anxiety or depression. The nightsweats continued and now she felt tired due to the sleep disruption, which in turn has started to affect her ability to work efficiently and be present for her family. The OB/GYN advised that for patients Sarah's age, she recommends oral birth control pills to help regulate cycles and moods. Wrapping up the appointment, she prescribed a low dose birth control pill.

Feeling unsatisfied and wanting to discuss all of her options, Sarah returned to social media, which directed her to The Menopause Society (TMS) website where she searched for a doctor that had been awarded

DOI: 10.4324/9781003632245-2

the credential of The Menopause Society Certified Practitioner (MSCP) (*Choosing a Healthcare Practitioner*, 2025). From there, Sarah found Dr. Naomi Busch, MD, MSCP at her practice Seattle Menopause Medicine and scheduled a visit.

Prior to the appointment, Sarah was asked to fill out the menopause checklist and realized that in addition to difficulty with sleep, fluctuating moods, and night sweats, she has also been having heart palpitations, difficulty with concentration and word finding, headaches, and joint pain. Sarah had not linked these symptoms to perimenopause at all. Dr. Busch had more time than most OB/GYNs or PCPs and was able to listen to her full story, collect past medical and family history, and come up with a comprehensive and personalized perimenopause plan. They discussed the benefits and risks of oral contraception as a way to level out the cycles, as many symptoms are influenced by the highs and lows of hormones. Combined hormonal contraception (CHC) helps with regulating the period, which in perimenopause can become irregular and sometimes heavy. It also provides contraception, which is necessary as at 44, Sarah can still become pregnant.

Sarah and Dr. Busch also discussed other options including progestin only pills, levonorgestrel intrauterine device (IUD), and menopausal hormone therapy (MHT). Sarah decided that since she still needed contraception and MHT does not provide this, she would like to move forward with a levonorgestrel IUD and also add an estradiol patch for her perimenopausal symptoms. She immediately felt more comfortable understanding the process and hoped that within a few months she would be feeling more like herself. Sarah also knew that if she continued to struggle, there were other options to explore. This gave her hope that there was a path forward, and when she left the appointment, she was already starting to feel better.

Thankfully, Sarah was informed enough to recognize the early stages of perimenopause, one of the good things that has come from "The Menopause Goldrush," a term used to describe the recent flood of menopause treatments and recommendations. The good news is that conversations about menopause are finally seeing the light of day. The bad news is that with all of the new information unfurling online at breakneck speed, it can be hard to discern between science and snake oil.

When it comes to menopause, there is still a lot we don't know, because historically, medical research has largely focused on men. There remains a major gap in understanding women's health. It's exciting to see menopause start to receive the attention it deserves, but letting the research naturally unfold will require having patience with the process.

WHAT'S MY FIRST STEP?

The Menopause Society, the preeminent organization leading the conversation about improving women's health, suggests that when a woman like Sarah suspects she's in perimenopause, it is an excellent time to have a complete medical examination. A qualified healthcare professional can also test for other causes of symptoms that can mimic perimenopause, such as thyroid disease or diabetes. Later in this chapter, we'll address other possible reasons for irregular cycles. Otherwise, according to Nanette Santoro, MD, "If it's walking like a duck and quacking like a duck, and you have the appropriate aged woman who is having some menopausal symptoms, you really don't need to do testing" (Santoro, 2024).

The material in this chapter can be a little technical, but I hope you'll find it useful. Feel free to read it "buffet style," skipping around to the sections relevant to you, or heck, read the whole darn thing. Understanding the menopause transition, and the various biological events to look for, is central to this chapter. So let's get started!

The stage before perimenopause is called premenopause, which is the reproductive stage from the start of menarche until the first cycle irregularity (perimenopause). The three stages of menopause after this are: Perimenopause, menopause, and the post-menopause. The menopause transition is the term used to define the first sign of cycle irregularity all the way until the final menstrual period (FMP). This term is often interchanged with the more popular term perimenopause, which means "around menopause". Technically speaking, perimenopause also starts at the first sign of cycle irregularity, but ends one year *after* the FMP. The median age of the onset of the menopause transition is 47 years old. This first stage is called early perimenopause, and there can be an irregularity of period by seven or more days, or a skipped period. There are patients who still have regular cycles that don't meet this criteria but still have perimenopausal symptoms; usually menstrual changes aren't far behind. Late perimenopause has a median age of 49 years old. The marker for late perimenopause is amenorrhea (absence of a menstrual cycle) for 60 days or more. Late perimenopause tends to have more characteristic "menopausal" symptoms such as hot flashes and night sweats, as estrogen levels get lower and the FMP draws nearer. Early perimenopause usually lasts longer than late perimenopause. The median age for menopause is 51-52 years old in most countries.

The most common symptom, occurring in approximately 70 percent of women, is vasomotor symptoms (VMS). Hot flashes and night sweats are terms used under the umbrella of VMS. They can be mild, moderate, or severe. VMS also vary by race and ethnicity. In the Journal of The Menopause Society article *Basics of Vasomotor Symptoms,* author Dr. Rebecca Thurston says, "The Study of Women's Health Across the Nation (SWAN) shows that U.S. Black women will be most likely to get VMS and have the most persistent, frequent, and bothersome VMS of any racial/ethnic group; however, most women across the racial/ethnic groups studied (White, Black, Chinese, Japanese, Latina/Hispanic) experienced VMS during menopause" (Thurston, 2024).

The second most common symptom of perimenopause is interrupted sleep, and the third most bothersome symptom is mood disruption. Of course these have a bi-directional effect, in which each of the symptoms can impact and intensify the other.

A menstrual calendar is a useful tracking tool to let you know where you stand in the menopause transition. The idea is to track your menstrual pattern so you have a heads up about where you are on your journey and what symptoms to look for. There are many ways to track your cycle – from pen and paper to apps on your phone. The key is finding a method that will be useful to you *and* protect your data.

The Basics of Menopause

Menopause marks an important stage in a woman's life, characterized by changes in bleeding patterns, hormone levels, body composition, and psychological well-being (Crandall, 2023, p. 1).

- Premenopause is the reproductive stage between the start of menarche and the start of perimenopause.
- Early perimenopause is characterized by irregular menstrual cycle changes in the length of time between periods (seven or more days persistent difference in cycle lengths from previous normal cycle). The most common age of onset for perimenopause is 47.
- Late perimenopause is marked by 60 or more days of amenorrhea. The median age is 49 years old.
- Perimenopause is the time from the onset of cycle irregularity until 12 months after the FMP.
- The menopause transition (MT) is defined as the time from the onset of cycle irregularity until the time of the FMP.
- Natural menopause is marked by the permanent cessation of menstrual periods for 12 months. Occurrence of natural menopause can only be determined retroactively after 12 consecutive months of amenorrhea, after the FMP. The most common age of the FMP is 51.5, in high-income countries.
- Early menopause is menopause before age 45.
- Menopause is usually considered late when it occurs after age 54.
- Postmenopause starts 12 months after the FMP.
- Early postmenopause is the stage within eight years of the FMP, otherwise it's classified as late postmenopause.
- Surgical menopause is the removal of both ovaries (called a bilateral oophorectomy) before you've gone through a natural menopause, causing sudden onset of menopause.
- Primary Ovarian Insufficiency (POI) is the cessation of ovarian function before the age of 40 (also referred to as premature ovarian insufficiency, as well as premature menopause).

WHAT IF I'M ON BIRTH CONTROL?

Dr. Amy Voedisch, an OB/GYN, MSCP at Stanford University who specializes in contraception and menopause believes there are benefits to being on contraception in the perimenopause phase. The main culprit causing perimenopausal symptoms is hormonal fluctuations. Our

Table 1.1 Acronym Glossary

Term	*Acronym*
Combined hormonal contraception	CHC
Conjugated equine estrogen	CEE
Designated female at birth	DFAB
Ethinyl estradiol	EE
Estrogen plus progesterone therapy	EPT
Estrogen therapy	ET
Final menstrual period	FMP
Follicle-stimulating hormone	FSH
Gender-affirming hormone therapy	GAHT
Genitourinary syndrome of menopause	GSM
Hormone replacement therapy	HRT
Hormone therapy	HT
Hypoactive sexual desire disorder	HSDD
Levonorgestrel intrauterine device	IUD
Menopause hormone therapy	MHT
Menopause transition	MT
Oral contraceptive pills	OCP
Polycystic ovary syndrome	PCOS
Primary ovarian insufficiency	POI
Progestin only pills	POP
Stellate ganglion block	SGB
The Menopause Society	TMS
The Menopause Society Certified Practitioner	MSCP
Transgender and gender diverse	TGD
Vasomotor symptoms	VMS
Women's Health Initiative Study	WHI

ovaries are trying to ovulate every month and signals from our brain control ovarian hormonal production. In perimenopause, our ovaries are slowing down. Some months they can overproduce hormones and other months they may not be able to respond to all the brain signals. This causes changes in levels of hormones in our bodies, mainly estradiol – a type of estrogen. We have estrogen receptors everywhere, with a large concentration in our brains. When estradiol levels rise and fall abruptly, this is very disruptive to our bodies, especially our brains, and can lead to many of the symptoms detailed below. Some birth control methods suppress ovarian function and can help relieve these symptoms by stabilizing our hormone levels. No more fluctuations can equal less symptoms! If your doctor suggests birth control as an option for your symptoms, this is a reasonable approach to consider.

Although our ovaries are slowing down, they do still release eggs and conception can occur. It is a common misconception that you can't get pregnant during perimenopause. Until you go a full 12 months without bleeding and are officially in menopause, you can still get pregnant. This is why TMS recommends contraception until you are in menopause or reach age 55.

When we talk about birth control, what do we mean? There are many options and it can be confusing to know what options might help in perimenopause and what options won't. Let's dig into the possibilities here.

- Birth control pills aka oral contraceptive pills (OCPs)

When we mention birth control pills, we often mean combined hormonal contraceptive pills (CHC). These pills contain both an estrogen and a progestin. These two substances work together to suppress ovarian function (your ovaries do not ovulate and hormonal production is low) and result in lighter, less painful, and more predictable periods. These combination pills can be helpful in perimenopause. They can control wonky bleeding and the estrogen in these pills, called ethinyl estradiol, can help with other symptoms such as joint pain, mood fluctuations, and cognition. There are times when ethinyl estradiol doesn't cut it and symptoms can occur even if you are using these combination products. If that happens to you, it's time to think about different medications to control your symptoms. There are other combined hormonal contraceptive options such as a patch and a vaginal ring that work similarly and contain similar products to the oral pills.

- Progestin only pills (POPs)

There are also pills that do not contain an estrogen and only contain a progestin. One type contains a progestin called norethinedrone and provides birth control but does not work by suppressing ovulation. It instead increases our cervical mucus and forms a barrier against sperm. The other oral progestin pill contains drospirenone, which does suppress ovulation and can be helpful to control perimenopausal symptoms by flattening estradiol fluctuations.

- Intrauterine devices (IUD)

IUDs are highly effective methods of contraception that can last three to ten years depending on the device used. There are two general types of intrauterine devices. One type contains the progestin levonorgestrel, with three different doses available in the United States. These devices do a great job of controlling bleeding but do not impact ovarian function or other hormone levels. The other type of IUD is a copper IUD. These do not contain any hormones and can lead to heavier periods for some women. They have no impact on perimenopausal symptoms.

- Contraceptive implant

The contraceptive implant contains a progestin and is inserted in the arm under the skin. It does suppress ovulation and generally results in lighter and shorter bleeding. It may help with some perimenopausal symptoms.

- Contraceptive injection

There is a progestin-only injection that can be given every three months to suppress ovulation called Depo Provera. The injection generally results in either no bleeding or very light periods. Given its impact on bleeding and ovarian hormone production, perimenopausal symptoms may be lessened on the injection.

Although some contraception can mask perimenopausal symptoms, some women become symptomatic while taking birth control. They may be dismissed (i.e. you can't have symptoms, you are on birth control pills!) but this means it's time to change up your hormonal medication!

We are often asked, "How will I know if I am in perimenopause or menopause if I am on birth control?" There are some ways to tell. First, if you start having symptoms that is a solid indicator of your perimenopausal status. If you are on birth control pills but do not have a period during the placebo week that is another sign. We can also conduct lab testing to help us determine if perimenopause has begun. For example, on the birth control injection you can check hormone levels right before your next injection. You can also check levels on either type of the IUD. When we say "check hormone levels," we generally mean estradiol (the estrogen produced by the ovaries) and follicle stimulating hormone (FSH); this is the main signal from the brain that communicates with the ovaries. In menopause, estradiol is low and the FSH is high. In perimenopause both of these hormones fluctuate wildly, making it hard to interpret lab results. However, testing can be part of the puzzle when trying to determine the cause of symptoms.

It's important to understand that birth control does not change your timeline through perimenopause and menopause. You are programmed to go through that phase on your own unique timeline regardless of whether or not you are on birth control. Birth control can mask the symptoms but not alter the timeline.

When to Test Your Hormones?

Social media influencers often tout the importance of testing your hormone levels. Hormone levels can fluctuate wildly, especially during perimenopause. One day your levels will be normal, later they could be low, indicating menopause, and then a few weeks later sky high. This makes hormone testing unpredictable and not particularly useful. Here are instances in which hormone testing can be valuable.

- As part of an evaluation for irregular periods, especially when they are absent and spaced far apart. Irregular bleeding is common in women over age 40, in particular those over age 45, but irregular bleeding prior to this warrants a work-up. Irregular bleeding over age 40 also should be discussed with your health care professional to determine the appropriate evaluation.
- When your uterus has been removed surgically (medically known as a hysterectomy) and you can no longer use periods as an indicator for your ovarian function, it may be helpful to check labs to determine the approximate age of menopause.
- When you are on estrogen therapy but are still having symptoms, your estradiol level can be checked to ensure you are properly absorbing your medication. Otherwise hormone

levels are not routinely checked while on HT. Doses are usually titrated based on symptoms and side effects.

When should hormones NOT be checked?

- When you are taking CHC, your natural estradiol levels are suppressed. It can be difficult to test hormone levels with this medication. Sometimes you can take a short break (one to six weeks) from the CHC to check levels if indicated.
- Routinely as part of therapy management. There is no target level for therapy. Dosage is determined based on symptom control. The range for "normal" for estrogen therapy is wide and each individual will feel well at their own unique level.

THE MOST COMMON SYMPTOMS IN THE MENOPAUSE TRANSITION

Vasomotor Symptoms (VMS)

VMS are the most well known of the perimenopausal and menopausal symptoms. They are also called hot flashes if they happen during the day and night sweats when they occur at night. They are caused by overactivity of the thermostat in our brain. Estrogen helps to control the thermostat and keep it steady, but the changing and then ultimately low levels of estrogen in menopause leads to VMS. VMS typically begin with a warm feeling in the chest that radiates up the neck and into the head. It can result in profuse sweating. Chills can follow the sweating. These can be disruptive to sleep and your ability to concentrate and focus. The earlier in the menopause transition the onset of VMS, the longer they usually persist into menopause. Fortunately over 80 percent of women will have resolution of VMS by their mid-to-late 50s. Unfortunately 10–15 percent will be "super flashers" and continue to have symptoms into their 60s and beyond.

Genitourinary Syndrome of Menopause (GSM)

GSM describes the physical changes that occur in the genitourinary region due to low levels of estrogen. Although these symptoms can be present in perimenopause, they usually become more pronounced in menopause and beyond. It is one of the few symptoms of menopause that tends to worsen with time. The lack of estrogen causes a loss of collagen and elasticity in the tissues of the vagina, leading to a decrease in pliability that can cause pain with penetrative sexual activity. The lack of estrogen also leads to a decrease in lubrication, which can cause dryness, itching, or burning. There is also an increased risk of urinary tract infections. Topical local estrogen therapy in the vagina and vulva can relieve these symptoms.

Joint Pain: Arthralgia

Estrogen receptors in the joints respond to the changing estrogen levels with pain and stiffness. New onset joint pain is common during the menopause transition and does respond to estrogen therapy. For Asian women, physical symptoms such as body aches and joint pains, as well as psychological symptoms, are recognized to be more prevalent than VMS (Islam et al., 2015).

Mood, Cognitive Function, and Sleep

The bulk of estrogen receptors in our bodies are in the brain. The impact of estrogen on the brain cannot be overstated. Changing estrogen levels can lead to not only VMS but also mood changes. Irritability, depression, and anxiety are common and may be debilitating. Estrogen therapy can be as beneficial as antidepressants in perimenopausal women with mood changes (Horst et al., 2025).

The brain fog of menopause transition and menopause is concerning and leads many to worry about the early onset of dementia. Dementia in women under age 65 is rare, but difficulty concentrating, word finding issues, and easy distractibility are some of the common cognitive symptoms during this time. Women often also ask if they have a new onset of ADHD, as the symptoms feel similar and make it challenging to complete previously easy tasks at home or work. The brain fog of perimenopause can mimic ADHD traits and it's possible that ADHD is unmasked during this time as well. Evaluation with a psychiatrist who specializes in adult diagnosis of ADHD may be appropriate.

Sleep can be challenging as well. Usually women can fall asleep but wake at 2 a.m. and have difficulty falling back to sleep. This sleep disturbance is triggered by VMS, anxiety or depression, and poor sleep hygiene that finally "catches up with us." There can also be unmasking of an underlying sleep disorder (similar to ADHD above). Sleep apnea is common, presents differently, and is often underdiagnosed in women. A sleep clinic evaluation is reasonable if sleep disruptions do not improve with other therapies. See more on this in Chapter Three.

Migraines

Migraines can be triggered by drops in estrogen levels and can be particularly bothersome during perimenopause when estrogen can rise and fall precipitously. Stabilizing estrogen levels with combined hormonal contraception or MHT can be therapeutic.

Bone Loss

Estrogen is a bone builder and helps to maintain and increase our bone density. Our bone mass peaks in our 30s, with a slow decline until perimenopause and menopause, where the rate of bone loss accelerates. Estrogen is an approved therapy for low bone mass (osteopenia) and the prevention of osteoporosis.

MOST COMMON TREATMENTS

The term hormone therapy (HT) has replaced the former term hormone replacement therapy (HRT), because you are "adding hormones" to a level that will make you feel better. HT is the use of hormones to treat perimenopausal and menopausal symptoms. The goal of HT is to supplement with enough hormones that symptoms are improved but not so much that you are "replacing" hormones back to their premenopausal levels. We don't need estradiol levels that high at this stage in our lives.

HT usually involves an estrogen component and, if you have a uterus, a progestogen as well. Why do you need a progestogen if you have a uterus? The estrogen can stimulate the lining of the uterus to grow and we need progestogen to counterbalance this effect; otherwise, it can lead to overgrowth, precancer and/or cancer, and cause irregular bleeding.

HT can mean many different things. If you are in perimenopause, it may mean combined hormonal contraception or the combination of a progestin only contraceptive such as the oral pill or IUD with separate estrogen therapy. If you are in menopause it may mean estrogen therapy with a progesterone to counterbalance the effects of the estradiol – but not necessarily birth control. This is also often referred to as menopausal hormone therapy (MHT) and can also be used in perimenopause in those that do not need or desire contraception. The point of all hormonal methods is to try to provide the body with a stable, steady state of estrogen to minimize symptoms.

Types of Hormone Therapy

The main component of HT is estrogen. In perimenopause, fluctuating levels of estradiol can wreak havoc on our bodies and minds, and in menopause, low levels of estradiol lead to symptoms of estrogen depletion. Estrogen therapy can come in different forms.

- Estradiol. This is similar to what our ovaries normally make and is often called "bio-identical." Bio-identical is a marketing term that was coined after the WHI study (detailed below) to try to denote a safer option with lower risks. All estrogen and progestogen products have risks and being "bio-identical" does not mean it is better or safer than other products on the market. That being said, estradiol is the most popular option for estrogen therapy. It is available in transdermal routes such as a patch, gel or spray, in oral pills, and vaginal creams, suppository and a ring.
- Conjugated equine estrogen (CEE) is one of the oldest estrogen products available and is often marketed under the trade name "Premarin." It is available in an oral form pill or a vaginal cream. There is controversy around the manufacturing of CEE, as it is collected from the urine of pregnant mares and the treatment of the horses is questionable at best.
- Estetrol is a new estrogen that is currently only available in combination with drospirenone as a birth control pill, but is under investigation as a combination and stand-alone product for menopausal therapy. It is expected to reach the market soon. As a birth control option it is an excellent choice for those patients who have symptoms with traditional pills containing ethinyl estradiol.
- Ethinyl estradiol (EE). Although usually used in combined contraceptives, there are also products available in menopausal dosing

containing ethinyl estradiol. These are safe but rarely used due to the availability and popularity of estradiol.

Progestogens are the other hormones contained in HT. Progestogens can be either progesterone or progestins.

- Progesterone is similar to the progesterone made by our ovaries and is also considered "bio-identical." It is available in an oral form only and is not a contraceptive. Progesterone protects the lining of the uterus from estrogen and can be helpful for sleep issues, as it has a mild sedative effect.
- Progestins are molecules that work at the progesterone receptor and are usually found in contraceptive products either in combination with an estrogen or as stand-alone products. There are also oral products that can be combined with an estrogen and used as part of HT.
- There are combination oral pills and transdermal patches that contain an estrogen and a progestogen together. The transdermal products contain estradiol and a progestin while the oral products come in a variety of combinations.

What Should I Do if I Am Having Symptoms while Taking a Contraceptive?

This is a frequent question and it depends on the contraceptive you are using.

- Combined hormonal birth control such as a pill, patch, or ring.

If you are having symptoms while taking a combined contraceptive you can switch to a method that contains a different type of estrogen than ethinyl estradiol. The estetrol containing contraceptive is a reasonable option and there are limited options of CHC that contain estradiol. Alternatively, you can change to a progestin only contraceptive and combine it with estradiol therapy to treat perimenopausal symptoms and provide contraception. If you do not need contraception, then traditional MHT is a reasonable approach as well.

- Progestin only contraceptives can be combined with estradiol if perimenopausal symptoms develop.
    - The progestin IUD has been well studied in combination with estrogen therapy to treat perimenopausal and menopausal symptoms. The highest dosed and most popular device can safely be used for five years.
    - The progestin injection route has not been studied as extensively as its oral counterpart for MHT, but the medication is highly effective at protecting the uterus.
    - The implant has not been well studied in this setting and is not advised to be combined with estrogen therapy until more data are available.
    - Both oral POP options can be combined with estrogen therapy safely.

What Are the Benefits of MHT?

Besides treating bothersome symptoms and improving quality of life, there are some medical benefits to MHT, as well. MHT is approved for the prevention of osteoporosis in the United States and indicates a reduction in bone fractures and bone loss. Globally, MHT is approved for both prevention and treatment of osteoporosis. There is also a slight decrease in risk of colorectal cancer. And most impressively, MHT reduces the risk of cardiovascular disease and mortality rates in users.

There is a caveat to these benefits: MHT must be started within ten years of the final menstrual period and/or before age 60. If MHT is started later than this time frame, it can lead to an increase in cardiovascular disease, heart attacks, stroke, and dementia. Note these increased risks are associated with *when MHT is started*, not with continuation. There are some women who use MHT into their 70s and 80s and this is safe, as long as they started it in the earlier time frame and do not develop breast cancer, cardiovascular disease such as a stroke or heart attack, dementia, or a blood clot.

What Are the Risks of MHT?

There are some risks involved in MHT. Estrogens stimulate the lining of the uterus to grow, and if not properly protected with progestogen, can lead to precancer and cancers. Estrogen also slightly increases the risk of blood clots in the legs and lungs. This risk is higher with combined hormonal birth control containing ethinyl estradiol than with MHT, but still less than a one percent risk in healthy women.

You may have read or recall hearing about the WHI, or Women's Health Initiative Study, which was published in July 2002 (*Women's Health Initiative (Whi) | Nhlbi, Nih*, n.d.). Based on literature from the Women's Health Initiative (WHI), when estrogen was combined with progestogen (EPT), there was a small increase in getting breast cancer after five years of using EPT, with no increase in mortality. There was an increased risk of about one extra case per 1000 women every year, but even this has been questioned based on the data and confounding variables and additional research with women of varying ages (The British Menopause Society, 2020; Attia, 2025; Pinkerton, 2025). Additionally for the WHI, people with no uterus, who took only estrogen and no progestogen therapy, had no increased risk for breast cancer.

Prior to the WHI, MHT was used liberally and thought to be the "fountain of youth." The WHI was a large randomized control trial looking at the prevention of heart disease in users. During the course of the study, the researchers discovered that the risk of breast cancer was higher in MHT users. The study was abruptly stopped and the results splashed all over the news: MHT causes cancer!!! This led to extraordinary discontinuation of MHT and rates of use plummeted.

The most flawed part of this study was that it didn't start women in the study on their hormones until the average age of 63 (Chester et al., 2018). With an average age of menopause being 51.5, that means some of the women were given HT 12 years after their final menstrual period, when all of the circuitry and cells that would have responded to estrogen had gone away. Dr. Louann Brizendine, founder of the University of California, San Francisco (UCSF) Hormone Clinic explains, "It's like a lawn you don't water for 12 years – when you water a dead lawn nothing happens" (Darpinian, 2023).

It has been more than 20 years since that study and we now understand the window of opportunity for MHT. Meaning, when started around the time of menopause or before the age of 60, the benefits of MHT generally outweigh the risks. When starting more than ten years from menopause, the pendulum swings with the risk of stroke, heart attack, and dementia increasing. The risk of breast cancer stays the same regardless of time of initiation. We now have a more balanced, nuanced understanding of the risks and benefits of MHT.

After the WHI study and the resultant decline in MHT use, women suffered from terrible symptoms. Looking for an answer, the concept of "bio-identical" hormones arose. The WHI study used conjugated equine estrogen and an oral progestin called medroxyprogesterone. Bio-identical hormones, meaning estradiol and progesterone, were marketed as being safer options because they were "natural" and similar to what our ovaries already make. While it is true that estradiol and progesterone are similar to our normally produced hormones and they do a great job of controlling symptoms, they are not safer than the products used in the WHI study. All of these products are made in a lab, they are all synthetic and they are not "natural." This also applies to compounded hormonal medications. Compounded products are not regulated by the FDA and each prescription can vary from refill to refill, making it difficult to know exactly what you are receiving. Compounded products are also made from the basic synthetic chemicals that comprise the FDA products and are not safer; in fact, they may be less safe given the lack of regulation.

Who Should Avoid MHT?

There are situations in which MHT should be avoided due to risks. This includes women with a personal history of breast cancer. If you have the breast cancer gene or a family history of breast cancer, you are still a candidate for MHT. If you have a history of a blood clot in your legs or lung, a stroke, a heart attack, other estrogen dependent cancers or uncontrolled blood pressure, you should avoid MHT.

Should I Take MHT?

Whether a woman should or should not use MHT is beyond the scope of this book, and as always in such situations, the benefits of treating bothersome symptoms on a woman's quality of life must be weighed against the potential risks associated with MHT and should be discussed with a healthcare professional.

How Long Should I Take MHT?

This depends on your symptoms. For some women, symptoms resolve in their 50s and they are able to discontinue MHT. For others, symptoms persist well into their 60s and beyond. If you develop the contraindications listed above, you must stop MHT. Otherwise *there is no age at which you must stop* MHT. Many believe that because the WHI showed an increased risk of MHT in those who started in their 60s, this meant MHT should not be used after the age of 60 or 65. However those risks are for women who want to start MHT for the first time, *not* for those who started MHT earlier and want to continue. The decision to continue is a personal one between you and your health care physician or provider.

At the time of this publication, there are only four US Food and Drug Administration (FDA)-approved reasons for MHT: VMS, GSM, osteoporosis prevention, and early or premature menopause. Everything else is off label at this time. However, you do not need one of these reasons to start MHT, as data suggests it may be helpful for a plethora of other symptoms not listed above. Shared decision-making between patient and doctor is strongly encouraged when thinking about treating menopause symptoms. If you don't feel like you're getting the care you need, look in the TMS directory for a doctor with a MSCP certification.

Testosterone

Thanks to social media, testosterone is a buzz topic these days. Women are being encouraged to ask their doctors for this medication, which wellness influencers promise will give us energy, boost our sex drive, and help with muscle mass and body composition. Despite popular belief, testosterone levels do not dramatically drop during perimenopause and menopause (unless our ovaries are surgically removed). Some people may experience a slow and steady decline of testosterone levels as they age.

Although it is being touted as the new fountain of youth, testosterone is only medically indicated for hypoactive sexual desire disorder (HSDD), or low libido, as an adjunct to other therapies that address the complex etiologies of HSDD. There is a global position paper written by experts from around the world that supports the use of testosterone, given in normal female ranges, for HSDD (Davis et al., 2019).

While there is no FDA-approved testosterone for women, they recommend using pharmaceutical gels at 1/10 the male doses or when needed, compounded creams. The use of pellet therapy is not supported. Pellet therapy is when a medication like testosterone, estrogen or a combination of both are inserted under the skin. Once inserted, the pellet cannot be easily removed and will last up to 90 days or longer. Pellet dosing is often difficult to regulate and elevated levels are a possible issue. Serum testosterone levels need to be monitored while on therapy to ensure levels stay in the normal female range.

Testosterone supplementation does have risks. When out of the normal female range, it can cause a deepening of your voice, enlargement of the Adam's apple and clitoris enlargement. These side effects are not reversible. Common reversible side effects are acne, male pattern hair loss, and oily skin – these go away once the testosterone is stopped.

NONHORMONAL THERAPY OPTIONS

Some women can't or don't want to take hormone therapy to control their symptoms and want to know what other options exist to help with symptom relief. TMS published non-hormonal treatment guidelines to aid women in finding the right therapy. The therapies range from lifestyle approaches to medical interventions and medications ("NAMS Position Statement," 2023).

Lifestyle

Lifestyle approaches include everything from cooling measures, exercise, dietary changes, and supplements.

- Cooling measures
  - There are moisture-wicking pajamas and bed cooling systems to help prevent VMS. Data does not show a difference in objective frequency or severity of VMS with these measures, but women often report a subjective reduction in their symptoms.
- Exercise and yoga
  - Exercise and yoga have many benefits, but studies do not show that they result in a reduction in objective menopausal symptoms such as VMS. Both are advised for general health

and overall well-being but may not make a big impact on menopausal and perimenopausal symptoms.

- Dietary changes
  - While research is ongoing, there are patterns of eating that have been studied in relation to the symptoms and health changes of menopause (Cano et al., 2020). See more on "gentle nutrition in midlife," in Chapter Five.
- Supplements
  - According to The Menopause Society Position Statement, no supplements have shown to make a difference in perimenopausal and menopausal symptoms. Some supplements may provide a placebo effect, but there are a few that should be used with caution – if at all – given their potential health risks. These include black cohosh and dong quai ("NAMS Position Statement," 2023).

Medical Interventions

Medical interventions have been proven to help relieve bothersome symptoms, especially VMS. These include cognitive behavioral therapy, clinical hypnosis, and stellate ganglion block. Acupuncture may be helpful for other issues, but has not been proven in studies to be beneficial in the context of perimenopause and menopause.

- Cognitive behavioral therapy (CBT)
  - CBT has many proven benefits and will be reviewed in more detail in Chapter Three, with respect to sleep. CBT also has a place in treating VMS. It has been shown to significantly reduce the frequency and intensity of VMS.
- Clinical hypnosis
  - Clinical hypnosis has also shown benefit in reducing VMS.
- Stellate ganglion block (SBG)
  - The stellate ganglion is a group of neurons in the neck and blockade of this ganglion is used to treat several conditions including pain and bothersome VMS. It must be done in a specialist's office and repeated to maintain efficacy.

Medications

There are several prescription medications that can be used for therapy. Some are approved by the FDA specifically for the treatment of VMS, while others are used "off label."

- Antidepressants
  - Antidepressants have been shown to not only address mood concerns but also reduce VMS. There is one medication, Brisdelle, which is FDA approved specifically for VMS.
- Fezolinetant (Veozah) is a new class of FDA approved medications that targets the "thermostat" in the brain to control VMS. It is effective and a reasonable option for those with bothersome symptoms who cannot take MHT. It rarely causes liver issues and liver enzymes are checked periodically during the first year on the medication. A new medication in the same class, elinzanetant, is expected to be available in the near future and has shown to have an improvement in sleep and quality of life.
- Gabapentin
  - Gabapentin is a medication used to treat seizures and pain disorders that has shown at lower dose to reduce VMS and improve sleep. This is an off-label use and not an approved indication for gabapentin.
- Oxybutynin
  - Oxybutynin is a medication used to treat overactive bladder and has also been shown to reduce the frequency and severity of VMS. There are concerns about side effects, including dry mouth, low blood pressure, and cognitive impact so use of oxybutynin for VMS is low.

PREMATURE OVARIAN INSUFFICIENCY

Premature ovarian insufficiency (POI), also called premature menopause, is the onset of menopause before age 40. It is usually diagnosed by an absence of menses (called amenorrhea) and may be associated with perimenopausal symptoms. There are many causes of amenorrhea, but when other causes have been excluded and the lab tests are consistent with menopause (elevated FSH and low estradiol) then the diagnosis of POI is made.

POI can occur at any age and rarely can present before the onset of periods. More classically it is diagnosed in women in their 20s and 30s. The causes of POI are varied; sometimes it is related to our genetics or the use of certain medications such as chemotherapy agents, or it can be autoimmune. Other times the cause is unknown. When a diagnosis of POI is made, it is important to rule out other medical issues such as thyroid disease, diabetes, celiac disease, and underlying genetic conditions.

Women with POI are at risk of cardiovascular disease, osteoporosis, and dementia due to the prolonged levels of low estrogen. It is recommended they are treated with true hormone replacement therapy (HRT) that mimics average levels of estradiol in premenopause until the age of 50. At that time, they can change to MHT dosing or stop all their HRT.

Although POI results in low ovarian hormones and function, occasional ovulation may occur, especially in the first years after diagnosis. Women who are not interested in conception should be given a progestin contraceptive paired with estrogen therapy. CHC containing ethinyl estradiol is not recommended, as this type of estrogen isn't as beneficial for bone, brain, and cardiovascular health as estradiol.

IS IT PERIMENOPAUSE OR IS IT POLYCYSTIC OVARY SYNDROME?

by Julie Duffy Dillon, MS, RD, NCC, CEDS-C

After missing a few periods, you could be experiencing perimenopause or it could be something else. Medical issues cause cycle regularity and one diagnosis to keep in mind is Polycystic Ovary Syndrome, or PCOS. While PCOS is a common lifelong condition, it is easy for doctors to miss. It is a hormonal condition connected to trouble conceiving, insulin resistance, diabetes, and mood. Many healthcare providers think of PCOS only in the reproductive sense, yet it has lifelong metabolic and psychological consequences.

It is important to know if you have PCOS as you enter midlife, because these metabolic and psychological changes tend to worsen as one ages. You may feel extreme fatigue, carbohydrate cravings, intense depression or anxiety. Speak to your doctor if you have a history of irregular periods to rule out PCOS. A doctor will help you determine if you have PCOS by using the Rotterdam Criteria (Christ & Cedars, 2023). To be diagnosed, a person needs to meet 2 out of the 3 of these:

1. Irregular or absent periods
2. Signs of excess androgens, often referred to as "male hormones."
3. Evidence of multiple immature follicles (cysts) on at least one ovary.

Getting diagnosed with PCOS in midlife can be tricky, because a person needs to be able to conceive to meet the Rotterdam Criteria. If you are in peri or postmenopause, a doctor can help you get a diagnosis based on your period cycle history.

MIDLIFE PCOS

Going through midlife with PCOS will look different. Estrogen dipping during perimenopause looks like regular cycles for the first time in PCOS sufferers. Most people with PCOS complete menopause two to four years later than people without PCOS. When you've been used to heavy painful periods and anemia from blood loss, you may feel a sense of relief.

While the reproductive consequences of PCOS go away after menopause, the metabolic and psychological ones remain or worsen. That is why it is so important to get a proper PCOS diagnosis even in midlife. People with midlife PCOS tend to have worsened blood sugar, heart health, and sleep issues. Researchers note that midlife PCOS typically causes worsened mood with a higher likelihood of depression and anxiety.

Speak with your doctor if you are concerned about a missed PCOS diagnosis. You have the power to help improve your heart health and lower blood sugar. Here are some questions to bring up to your doctor to help you two decide if you have PCOS and ways to treat it:

- Review your menstrual history. How many cycles did you usually have per year? Were they irregular? Were they painful or heavy? Ask if you could meet criteria for PCOS based on this information.
- Check DHEA levels. This is an androgen that often remains high in midlife PCOS unlike testosterone.
- Ask to test your cholesterol panel including triglycerides, A1c (average blood sugar), and HOMA-IR (test to measure how much insulin is needed to normalize blood sugar,) since these all typically worsen with midlife PCOS.

- Consider a sleep study. Most people with PCOS have a sleep disorder, especially after midlife. Diagnosing and treating a sleep issue will help improve your heart health and blood sugar. It will also help you not feel so tired all the time!

TOP SIX TIPS FOR HEALTHY LIVING WITH PCOS

1. Be sure you are eating enough with three daily meals and snacks. Eating less in the short term may lower blood sugar, yet long term it does not. Long term studies show diets worsen health and deplete your energy.
2. Consider adding protein to your meals and snacks. Don't worry about taking anything away, rather focus on adding protein to see if it helps with your energy levels and mood. Doing this long term can help some people with PCOS lower insulin and blood sugar.
3. Experiment with adding an inositol supplement (Dillon, 2017). Always speak with your healthcare provider first. Inositol, when taken correctly, helps lower cholesterol, insulin, and blood sugar.
4. Make sure you are getting enough rest. Getting adequate sleep and taking breaks throughout the day can lower your inflammation and insulin levels. Rest through grounding exercises and meditation also help.
5. Connect with movement you enjoy. Don't worry about doing high intensity exercises unless you actually enjoy them. Be sure to eat enough to sustain yourself through them. Consistent lower intensity movement such as walking has been found to help with fatty liver disease, often seen in people with PCOS.
6. Avoid weight cycling. Going on and off diets worsens PCOS. Find ways to avoid dieting to help you avoid weight cycling.

SEX, GENDER, AND MENOPAUSE

by Dr. Abby Cobb-Walch

Everyone that has a uterus and ovaries will go through the menopause. But not everyone who traverses menopause identifies as female. Gender is a spectrum, and individuals designated female at birth (DFAB) who do not present or identify as female will experience menopause as well, including transgender men and non-binary individuals (see Table 1.2).

Table 1.2 Sex and Gender Definitions

Term	Definition
Sex	Characteristic designated at birth as either male or female, typically based on the appearance of the external genitalia
Gender	One's internal core sense of gender that is not binary, although most people identify as male (boy or man) or female (girl or woman)
Cisgender	Refers to people who have a gender aligning with their sex designated at birth
Gender incongruence	Term used when gender does not align with sex designated at birth
Gender dysphoria	Distress and unease experienced because of gender incongruence
Transgender and gender diverse (TGD)	Umbrella term used to describe a diverse group of people with gender incongruence

Gender-affirming medical care for transgender and gender diverse (TGD) people requires an individualized approach. Some TGD individuals do not require any medical or surgical interventions for affirmation of their gender, while others require gender-affirming hormone therapy (GAHT), surgical interventions, or both. Gender-affirming medical and surgical interventions are considered medically necessary for TGD individuals who wish to pursue them (Hembree et al., 2017; Coleman et al., 2022).

There are unique considerations for TGD individuals traversing menopause, a life event that typically centers on the experiences of cisgender women (Toze & Westwood, 2025). For TGD individuals DFAB, menopause may occur at various ages and/or stages of their gender journey, and co-occurrence of classical menopausal symptoms are dependent on whether GAHT and/or surgeries have been pursued (Toze & Westwood, 2025). TGD persons that do not initiate any GAHT, and therefore experience classic menopause at the same time as their cisgender female peers, may face unique challenges in having their needs understood and met by health care clinicians (Toze & Westwood, 2025).

GAHT for TGD persons DFAB typically involves testosterone therapy, which typically results in cessation of menstrual periods within six months (Hembree et al., 2017; Toze & Westwood, 2025; Kumar et al., 2022; Asseler et al., 2024). While having similarities to menopause experienced by cisgender women, TGD people may not view their experience in this way, and they are unlikely to experience classic symptoms of menopause that occur with estradiol suppression by continuing testosterone therapy (Toze & Westwood, 2025).

TGD persons DFAB may pursue various surgical procedures including hysterectomy (surgical removal of the uterus) with removal of both fallopian tubes with or without removal of one or both ovaries (Coleman et al., 2022; Carbonnel et al., 2021; Simko et al., 2024). GAHT is not a prerequisite for surgery; however, hormone therapy is advisable in individuals younger than age 50 years undergoing removal of both ovaries (bilateral oophorectomy) to prevent long-term adverse health effects of low sex hormones (Coleman et al., 2022). Potential benefits and risks of removing both ovaries at the time of hysterectomy must be discussed with patients given the potential impacts on fertility, bone health, cardiovascular health, neurocognitive status, oncologic risk, and endocrine management (Kumar et al., 2022; Carbonnel et al., 2021; Simko et al., 2024). Reasons to consider ovarian removal include 1) dysphoria associated with presence of ovaries, 2) personal/family history of increased ovarian cancer risk, and 3) avoidance of future ovarian disease (e.g., cyst, mass, cancer) (Coleman et al., 2022; Kumar et al., 2022; Simko et al., 2024; Grimstad et al., 2021).

Reasons to consider keeping the ovaries include 1) preservation of fertility, 2) "back-up" sex hormones (e.g., if patients lose access to hormone therapy), and 3) minimization of potential surgical risks (Kumar et al., 2022; Simko et al., 2024; Grimstad et al., 2021). Bilateral oophorectomy at the time of hysterectomy, or surgical menopause, in TGD individuals DFAB may or may not cause menopausal symptoms, depending on whether the individual is taking testosterone therapy (Simko et al., 2024).

A TRANSGENDER PERSPECTIVE

by Nik

As a youth, I was never the least bit in-tune with any of my biologically female experiences. I have no recollection of my first menstrual cycle, and my only memory of breast development involves a cousin's exclamation: "Nikki [my birth name], you finally have boobs!" I distinctly recall a sense of confusion – "I do? Oh, those. You certainly seem to imply that's a good thing. Am I supposed to care?"

The one thing I *do* recall was how much I absolutely despised my feminine voice and the genuine startle I experienced each time I heard it played back. It was not until much later in life that I began to understand why these were my experiences. It also illuminated why I had struggled so much with my body image over the years. I realized that I had never, ever identified with my female self. But after years of reflection and exploration, I came to terms with my gender identity. And in my thirties, I began my transition.

I began my medical transition with a bilateral mastectomy – referred to as "top surgery" by the transgender and non-binary community. (Myself, I much prefer the term "teetus deletus.") I immediately fell in love with my new chest and, for the first time, began to experience integration with my physical self. Post-surgery, I weighed more than I ever had in my life. Yet when I looked in the mirror, I loved what I saw. I loved the way I fit in my clothing. I had always blamed my weight for the discomfort I felt in my body, because that's what society told me was to blame. It must have been the extra pounds I carried around my gut, right? Turns out, I just hated my boobs. The more I became comfortable in my physical body, the more I recognized that I would never be able to exist comfortably with my voice as it was. I needed it to change. I accessed gender-affirming speech therapy, which helped me to alter things like pitch and prosody. However, I still sounded so much like a girl, and I was becoming paralyzingly self-conscious of speaking in unfamiliar settings. Enter gender-affirming hormone therapy.

Now that I had entered my integrated and self-aware era, I began to research gender-affirming hormone therapy (in my case, the use of testosterone to achieve male-associated secondary sex characteristics). I also began to reflect on my family's medical history. I recalled my mother's numerous emergency room visits when I was young, due to her unexplained heart palpitations and associated symptoms. It took years before a physician suggested she may be experiencing premature menopause. I remember my mother learning that my grandmother had also experienced premature menopause and a diagnosis of PCOS. This led me to reflect on my own teen years and young adulthood. I bled so irregularly, yet I never sought answers. When I say irregularly, I mean exceedingly irregularly – rarely monthly, mostly quarterly-ish, and sometimes...twice a year? My physician was aware, but she never suggested any interventions and, frankly, I didn't care. The less I bled, the better, as far as I was concerned. However as I have learned from my current health providers, this irregularity posed a health risk.

I began to wonder how menopause may, or may not, affect me as I considered gender-affirming hormone therapy. My Google searches provided limited information, and the reputable literature I did find failed to address menopause in transgender men. It was then I decided to connect with an endocrinologist.

I had so many questions. Most were specific to the gender-related changes I would experience on testosterone therapy. Most of these were desired – my voice would deepen, and I would sprout facial hair. Some were less desirable – I was informed that teenage acne would likely make a temporary but fierce comeback. I also had questions regarding how my personal and family history may interact with testosterone therapy. It was explained to me that, in a transgender individual maintaining their ovaries, testosterone therapy would suppress the ovaries' estrogen production. The higher the testosterone dose, the stronger the estrogen suppression. My endocrinologist reflected that, if I was on a high-enough dose of testosterone, it was possible I may not experience menopause symptoms later in life, as my body would have already adjusted to the decrease in estrogen. Given that I was pursuing a lower dosage and more of a balanced transition, I had questions about what that would look like. The feedback I received was that, though I was likely to experience some degree of menopausal symptoms, "actual results may vary." Regardless, I was ready. And let me tell you, gender-affirming hormone therapy is a blessing. Remember how I thought I had entered my integrated era? Well, now I had REALLY entered my integrated era. I was becoming even more myself.

Having already had two gender-affirming surgeries (my initial bilateral mastectomy and a follow-up "revision" to fine-tune the results), I had assumed I was done with surgeries. Two was plenty for me; I have quite a bit of medical anxiety, and anesthesia freaks me out. The further I progressed into my transition, I began to fine-tune my testosterone dose and find the "sweet spot" that supported my gender needs as well as my overall health. It was then that I realized I would experience breakthrough bleeding without further intervention, so I began to explore the idea of a gender-affirming hysterectomy. It was then that I connected with a gender-affirming gynecologist.

Again, I had so many questions. What type of hysterectomy was recommended? A partial, removing only the uterus? A full, removing both the uterus and the cervix? What organs did she recommend removing? Should I keep my ovaries? One? Both? Everyone's gender journey is different, and everyone must come to their own right answer with the guidance of informed physicians. My doctor and I determined that I would have a total hysterectomy, removing the uterus and cervix but leaving behind both ovaries. This would eliminate any menstrual cycles but allow me a hormonal "security blanket." The reason I chose to keep two ovaries? Another security blanket. If I ever lost function in one, I would have a backup. Many transgender individuals live with the worry of whether we will lose access to our gender-affirming hormone therapies as political climates shift. As a safeguard, I opted to keep my ovaries so that I would never be left without any sex hormones at all, which I know to pose serious health risks. I learned that, because I was retaining my ovaries, I would not experience the surgically-induced menopause that is often mentioned in the same breath as "hysterectomy." That was an added benefit. Traversing menopause in my late thirties, while raising two hormonal teenagers, did not sound like an exciting journey for our household. So here I am, a transmasculine person living in a body that is finally my own, living a life that is more fulfilling than I ever imagined, and curiously awaiting the time that is considered menopausal, to find out what, if any, symptoms I may have to navigate.

WHERE TO SEEK HELP

Dr. Cobb-Walch provides hormone therapy specialty consultation and management at the UCSF Gender Affirming Health Program. Dr. Cobb-Walch is an endocrinologist, a doctor that specializes in diagnosing and treating conditions that affect the endocrine system. Endocrinologists diagnose and treat conditions caused by hormone imbalances, and some specialize in providing gender-affirming hormone therapy to transgender and gender diverse patients. Additional resources for gender-affirming health care are cited in the resource section at the back of the book.

PREVENTATIVE CARE: MOVING FORWARD WITH MICRO GOALS

Now that you have a basic understanding of what menopause is (and what it isn't), I hope it will be less overwhelming to take that first step in moving forward with thoughtful and meaningful health care. Women in midlife carry numerous responsibilities – homemaking, jobs and careers, parenting, caregiving for parents, children, partners and even friends. The Menopause Society (TMS) states, "Women aren't procrastinating on their healthcare appointments, they literally don't have the time for them" (*Making Menopause Work*, 2025). One of the reasons women don't have time is because society has not traditionally prioritized their health. TMS has advocated for more "menopause responsive workplaces," and personal and public health priorities must shift in order to provide flexibility so that women can access healthcare. There exists an increased awareness of common diseases in midlife, but as we wait for the research to unfold in women's health – specifically in the menopause space – preventative care is essential. However, this can seem overwhelming, especially when it has been put off. This is why I suggest starting with micro goals.

Calibrating goals, especially in midlife when we can have many competing priorities, often leaves preventative health care near the bottom of the list. Imagine a bedroom that is a disheveled mess and needs cleaning. Every time you walk into the room with the intent of cleaning it, the mess is so overwhelming that you turn and walk right back out. This is an example of a macro goal – in other words, it's too big. Now imagine covering the entire room with a sheet, except for the dresser, and cleaning that one thing. This is an example of a micro goal.

The key is to identify and prioritize micro goals that align with your larger aspirations. For example, if your objective is to stay on top of your preventative health care each year, a micro goal would be to first break down the different appointments – a colonoscopy, a mammogram, and so on. By breaking down large goals into manageable, incremental tasks, it's easier to make progress without feeling overwhelmed

Where to begin? If you feel stuck, it may be a signal that your health goals are too big and need to be broken down into smaller parts that can be tackled in achievable chunks. When the brain becomes overwhelmed, it can panic and even freeze. Try asking yourself, "What is one thing I can do today?" This can be a balm on the brain and a way to move out of freeze mode. If your list of preventative care appointments feels too big, try honing in on one thing as a manageable starting point – for example, if you need multiple tests, prioritize scheduling one at a time, or one each day/week.

This week I am going to look for my referral slip to get a colonoscopy, and call to schedule. That's it! Just the colonoscopy this week. Next week, I'll tackle something else.

Science has informed us that the more calibrated the goal, the better the outcome. Micro goals give us a sense of accomplishment and self mastery, both of which support taking on the next challenge (Darpinian, 2021).

MIDLIFE MICRO GOALS EXPLORATION

What micro goals would you set for yourself in the next two hours? The next 24 hours?

Women can have multiple healthcare providers, someone for primary care, another for gynecological care, and still others for specific specialty care. This can be confusing and difficult to navigate. It's okay to ask questions and request clarity. Hopefully, the content in this book helps you define and prioritize questions so that you can discuss your health needs with your medical team. It's your body and if you don't understand why something is happening or not happening, you deserve thorough and accessible answers.

It's important to know what the preventative health recommendations are as we age. Women need specific screening tests, preventative services, and procedures at different ages. A primary care provider is your first line for information. Depending on the specialty care you are receiving, engage your specialist to ask about prevention goals and any recommended care at certain ages. It's important to be an advocate for yourself and your own health. Unfortunately, this can seem or actually be intimidating, but that begs the question, "If you don't do it, who will?" After reading this chapter, I hope you are informed and empowered and equipped to be your best advocate.

By midlife, we have accumulated life experience that leads to wisdom. We are better at listening to ourselves and honoring our instincts. This can make the menopause transition a confusing one, because our signals change without warning, and no one tells us what we're supposed to be listening to. For example, as you saw in the preface, my pain was now physiological; the specialists and strategies I'd drawn on in the past no longer addressed my symptoms. My joint pain, the byproduct of hormonal fluctuation, was something I'd never experienced before. When the body starts speaking a different language, it's tempting to ignore the signals and use the same approaches that have always worked for us. But the search for *well-being* is informed by the new way things are unfolding.

Menopause is a normal process that is supposed to happen. Every woman who survives the middle age stage of life will go through menopause between ages 40–58. In the United States, female life expectancy is 81.2 – unchanged since 2012. With an increase in life expectancy, 40 percent of women's lives will be lived in post menopause. Experiences and treatments during this stage of life are as unique as each individual. Some people have very few symptoms, and some people have myriad symptoms, but physiologically the same things are happening to everyone.

Now you understand the nature of the menopause transition, know what symptoms to look for, and are familiar with some of the most common types of treatment. Knowledge is power. You are the authority of you, and being "menopause informed" is going to ground you in the options available to you when navigating this natural stage of life.

As we move into the next chapter to talk about changing bodies in midlife, you'll notice a weight-inclusive approach there and throughout the book, which puts an emphasis on viewing health and well-being as multifaceted, while directing efforts toward improving health behaviors such as sleep, social-emotional well-being, movement, attuned eating, and healthy relationships.

REFERENCES

Asseler, J. D., Del Valle, J. S., Chuva De Sousa Lopes, S. M., Verhoeven, M. O., Goddijn, M., Huirne, J. A. F., & Van Mello, N. M. (2024). One-third of amenorrheic transmasculine people on testosterone ovulate. *Cell Reports Medicine*, 5(3), 101440. https://doi.org/10.1016/j.xcrm.2024.101440

Attia, P. (2025, May 12). #348 – *Women's sexual health, menopause, and hormone replacement therapy (Hrt) | Rachel Rubin, M.D.* Peter Attia. https://peterattiamd.com/rachelrubin/

Cano, A., Marshall, S., Zolfaroli, I., Bitzer, J., Ceausu, I., Chedraui, P., Durmusoglu, F., Erkkola, R., Goulis, D. G., Hirschberg, A. L., Kiesel, L., Lopes, P., Pines, A., van Trotsenburg, M., Lambrinoudaki, I., & Rees, M. (2020). The Mediterranean diet and menopausal health: An EMAS position statement. *Maturitas*, 139, 90–97. https://doi.org/10.1016/j.maturitas.2020.07.001

Carbonnel, M., Karpel, L., Cordier, B., Pirtea, P., & Ayoubi, J. M. (2021). The uterus in transgender men. *Fertility and Sterility*, 116(4), 931–935. https://doi.org/10.1016/j.fertnstert.2021.07.005

Chester, R. C., Kling, J. M., & Manson, J. E. (2018). What the Women's Health Initiative has taught us about menopausal hormone therapy. *Clinical Cardiology*, 41(2), 247–252. https://doi.org/10.1002/clc.22891

Christ, J. P., & Cedars, M. I. (2023). Current guidelines for diagnosing pcos. *Diagnostics*, 13(6), 1113. https://doi.org/10.3390/diagnostics13061113

Choosing a Healthcare Practitioner. (2025). The Menopause Society. Retrieved May 23, 2025, from https://menopause.org/patient-education/choosing-a-healthcare-practitioner

Coleman, E., Radix, A. E., Bouman, W. P., Brown, G. R., De Vries, A. L. C., Deutsch, M. B., Ettner, R., Fraser, L., Goodman, M., Green, J., Hancock, A. B., Johnson, T. W., Karasic, D. H., Knudson, G. A., Leibowitz, S. F., Meyer-Bahlburg, H. F. L., Monstrey, S. J., Motmans, J., Nahata, L., … Arcelus, J. (2022). Standards of care for the health of transgender and gender diverse people, version 8. *International Journal of Transgender Health*, 23(sup1), S1–S259. https://doi.org/10.1080/26895269.2022.2100644

Crandall, C. (2023). *Menopause practice: A clinician's guide* (6th ed.). North American Menopause Society.

Darpinian, S. (2021, February 2). Why hope is so important in 2021. *Therapy Rocks!* Retrieved May 23, 2025, from https://audioboom.com/posts/7788973-why-hope-is-so-important-in-2021

Darpinian, S. (2023, September 29). The menopause brain and beyond. *Therapy Rocks!* Retrieved May 23, 2025, from https://audioboom.com/posts/8376467-the-menopause-brain-and-beyond

Davis, S. R., Baber, R., Panay, N., Bitzer, J., Cerdas Perez, S., Islam, R. M., Kaunitz, A. M., Kingsberg, S. A., Lambrinoudaki, I., Liu, J., Parish, S. J., Pinkerton, J., Rymer, J., Simon, J. A., Vignozzi, L., & Wierman, M. E. (2019). Global consensus position statement on the use of testosterone therapy for women. *Climacteric: The Journal of the International Menopause Society*, 22(5), 429–434. https://doi.org/10.1080/13697137.2019.1637079

Dillon, J. (2017, October 12). *Inositol*. Julie Duffy Dillon. https://julieduffydillon.com/inositol/

Grimstad, F., Boskey, E. R., Taghinia, A., & Ganor, O. (2021). Gender-affirming surgeries in transgender and gender diverse adolescent and young adults: A pediatric and adolescent gynecology primer. *Journal of Pediatric and Adolescent Gynecology*, 34(4), 442–448. https://doi.org/10.1016/j.jpag.2021.03.014

Hembree, W. C., Cohen-Kettenis, P. T., Gooren, L., Hannema, S. E., Meyer, W. J., Murad, M. H., Rosenthal, S. M., Safer, J. D., Tangpricha, V., & T'Sjoen, G. G. (2017). Endocrine treatment of gender-dysphoric/gender-incongruent persons: An endocrine society* clinical practice guideline. *The Journal of Clinical Endocrinology & Metabolism*, 102(11), 3869–3903. https://doi.org/10.1210/jc.2017-01658

Horst, K., Cirino, N., & Adams, K. E. (2025). Menopause and mental health. *Current Opinion in Obstetrics & Gynecology*, 37(2), 102–110. https://doi.org/10.1097/GCO.0000000000001014

Islam, M. R., Gartoulla, P., Bell, R. J., Fradkin, P., & Davis, S. R. (2015). Prevalence of menopausal symptoms in Asian midlife women: A systematic review. *Climacteric*, 18(2), 157–176. https://doi.org/10.3109/13697137.2014.937689

Kumar, S., Mukherjee, S., O'Dwyer, C., Wassersug, R., Bertin, E., Mehra, N., Dahl, M., Genoway, K., & Kavanagh, A. G. (2022). Health outcomes associated with having an oophorectomy versus retaining one's ovaries for transmasculine and gender diverse individuals treated with testosterone therapy: A systematic review. *Sexual Medicine Reviews*, 10(4), 636–647. https://doi.org/10.1016/j.sxmr.2022.03.003

Making Menopause Work. (2025). The Menopause Society. https://menopause.org/workplace

NAMS Position Statement. (2023). *The 2023 nonhormone therapy position statement of The North American Menopause Society*. The Menopause Society. https://menopause.org/wp-content/uploads/professional/2023-nonhormone-therapy-position-statement.pdf

Pinkerton, J. (2025). Hormone therapy. *Menopause Step-by-Step*, 32(1), 95–97. https://menopause.org/wp-content/uploads/professional/Pinkerton-Step-by-Step-Article.pdf

Santoro, N. (2024, October 30). *Menopause step by step | professional resources*. The Menopause Society. https://menopause.org/professional-resources/step-by-step

Simko, S., Popa, O., & Stuparich, M. (2024). Gender affirming care for the minimally invasive gynecologic surgeon. *Current Opinion in Obstetrics & Gynecology*, 36(4), 301–312. https://doi.org/10.1097/GCO.0000000000000956

The British Menopause Society. (2020). *BMS & WHC's 2020 recommendations on hormone replacement therapy in menopausal women*. g.uk/wp-content/uploads/2023/10/02-BMS-ConsensusStatement-BMS-WHC-2020-Recommendations-on-HRT-in-menopausal-women-SEPT2023-A.pdf

Thurston, R. C. (2024). Basics of vasomotor symptoms. *Menopause*, 31(12), 1085–1086. https://doi.org/10.1097/GME.0000000000002479

Toze, M., & Westwood, S. (2025). Experiences of menopause among non-binary and trans people. *International Journal of Transgender Health*, 26(2), 447–458. https://doi.org/10.1080/26895269.2024.2389924

Women's health initiative (Whi) | nhlbi, nih. (n.d.). https://www.nhlbi.nih.gov/science/womens-health-initiative-whi

What to Expect When Your Body Is Changing

Two

Physiologically our body is trying to help us, but society isn't along for this ride. It's time to re-educate society on what women's bodies are supposed to look like, and what's normal.

– Dr. Amy J Voedisch, OB/GYN, MCSP

I remember noticing body changes in what I realize now was late perimenopause. As a body image and eating disorder specialist for 25 years, I am fortunate to have enough body image resilience that the aesthetic changes to my body didn't disconcert me too much. Unfortunately, this is not the case for most women. In this chapter, we'll spend some time explaining some of the reasons biological females' bodies change in midlife, but will go into much more detail about how that impacts body image in Chapter Six.

CHANGING BODIES

When I interviewed registered dietitian (RD), and The Menopause Society Certified Practitioner (MSCP) Val Schonberg, she said, "Women are so inundated with diet culture that it's no longer enough to tell them to 'love their body.' They want to know WHY they are experiencing their body changes" (Darpinian, 2023a). I see this in the work I do with women as well, and find it interesting that understanding the physiology of the body can be helpful for creating some distance from the feelings that come up around body changes.

Menopause is a time when our body decides to redistribute our fat–and it likes to put our fat cells around our midsection. This physiological change happens because our ovaries are not making estrogen, and we need to get estrogen from other places, one of which is our fat cells, in particular the fat around our abdomens. These fat cells make a slightly

DOI: 10.4324/9781003632245-3

> different estrogen, but it's still an estrogen nonetheless. Estrogen is so important for all of our different body systems to run, so the estrogen coming from these new fat cells is what's helping to grease the wheels and help these different body systems to work.
>
> (Darpinian, 2023b)

Said Dr. Voedisch, OB/GYN, MCSP, "Physiologically our body is trying to help us, but society isn't along for this ride. It's time to re-educate society on what women's bodies are supposed to look like, and what's normal." And of course we can't talk about weight gain or weight redistribution in the menopause transition without also talking about aging. Schonberg says in her blog *The Weight of Menopause*, "First is the natural loss of lean tissue (muscle) that occurs as we get older. The body also becomes resistant to building muscle as we age (called anabolic resistance). Consequently, women may experience reduced muscle strength and may be less physically active and possibly with less intensity" (Schonberg, 2023).

As you can imagine, gaining weight is the number one concern expressed by most women. Dr. Naomi Busch notes that patients in the menopause transition ask her the same questions almost daily: "I've changed absolutely nothing, and I've gained X pounds. What can I do?"

The following is a short vignette from a visit with Dr. Busch, who believes in taking a weight inclusive approach that focuses on symptoms, concerns, and diagnosis rather than size. Natasha, a 49-year-old woman visited Seattle Menopause Medicine to see Dr. Busch, stating she "just does not feel like herself." She has concerns about weight gain, noting that she has not changed any of her normal activities. She continues to run three to four days a week and walks with friends most days. She reports that she eats healthy with lean meat, vegetables, and carbs. She feels like she is going crazy because none of clothes fit around the belly and she continues to gain weight. Recently, she has been hearing and seeing a lot of social media influencers talk about the value of fasting and wonders if she should try this to help her lose weight.

Natasha fills out a menopause checklist which is notable for disrupted sleep, joint pain, headaches, and hot flashes/night sweats.

Dr. Busch starts the conversation by first highlighting the other symptoms that Natasha did not mention. She asks about sleep, and it turns out that while falling asleep is not a problem, Natasha wakes up every night around 2 or 3 a.m. drenched in sweat. She also has to get up to urinate at least twice a night. Her husband reports that he thinks she may have started snoring. Her joint pain started a few years ago and she went to her primary care physician (PCP), who ran tests for inflammation. Everything was normal. Her joint pain tends to be worse in the morning but can happen throughout the day. At its worst, it can manifest in all of her joints and she had assumed this was just something she'd have to live with.

When discussing weight, Dr. Busch is careful to ask permission to discuss in detail what is happening with weight, nutrition, and movement. She also explains that it is normal to gain weight throughout our lives. The rate of weight gain is subtle – around 0.3–0.5 pounds per year – but during the transition through perimenopause and into early menopause the rate of weight gain may increase. For some it can be up to 2 pounds per year and others less, with the average around 1.5 pounds per year. There is also a noticeable body composition change with loss of lean body mass (muscle) and increase in central body fat (abdominal). The theory of why this happens is that the body starts to preferentially lay down fat, as fat can produce a form of estrogen called estrone, that while weaker than estradiol, can still supply much needed estrogen to our bodies. When estrogen (estradiol) is used in menopausal hormone therapy, it can signal the body that there is no need to store extra fat and it may lead to some reversal of this metabolic process. However, it does not lead to weight loss.

Dr. Busch cautions against dieting, since we know that this leads to a further reduction in metabolic rate as the body tries to defend itself from starvation. What is more important is changing some of our behaviors. We can start to lift weights – emphasizing lifting heavier weights with less reps rather than lower weights with more reps. We can build balanced plates that include sufficient protein to support our muscles before and after exercise. And we can rest our bodies by working on sleep hygiene, including our evening habits and sleep disruptions.

Dr. Busch suggests working with a weight-inclusive/anti-diet registered dietician who is familiar with menopause, as well as a private trainer to learn how to lift (if this is accessible). She also suggests a sleep study, as women in menopause transition can experience an increase in sleep apnea, leading to fatigue and other troubles. Finally, they have a discussion about hormone and non-hormonal therapy for hot flashes and night sweats to see if this fits with Natasha's goals.

CHANGING HAIR

When we hear the term body changes, we think about the body only, but in this particular phase of life, body image concerns include hair and skin, in addition to body composition.

If you had big hair coming of age in the 80s like I did, you are probably somewhere in the menopause transition right now. And if your big hair isn't very big anymore, it can take an unexpected toll on your body image, especially if it's a form of creative expression for you.

My type of hair loss is one of the two most common types for women during and after the menopause transition. It's called Female Pattern Hair Loss (FPHL) – medically known as *female androgenetic alopecia*. It's related to genetics and/or age-related hormone changes. This type of hair loss is a gradual thinning of hair over time, mainly on the crown of the head with widening through the center part. It can be alarming at first to see space in between hairs and your scalp peeking out in places it didn't before. Thinning hair is the first sign as the hair follicles become smaller, which makes the hair strands finer (Godman, 2023). The only FDA-approved treatment for FPHL is topical minoxidil (aka Rogaine for women), which comes in a foam that you apply daily to the crown of the scalp. It's affordable, over-the-counter, and kind of messy.

The second most common type of hair loss is a sudden onset of hair shedding, medically known as *telogen effluvium* (TE). According to *Menopause Practice: A Clinician's Guide* (6th Edition), "TE is a disruption of the hair cycle that occurs several months after a major life stressor or because of a chronic illness or prescribed medications known to promote hair loss such as anticoagulants and beta-blockers" (Crandall, 2023 p. 34). This type of hair loss often corrects on its own after the underlying cause is cured, but it can often coexist with FPHL, so if it does not remit on its own you would need to talk to your doctor about assessing for FPHL.

Not everyone will experience hair loss in midlife, but those who do may feel helpless and unsure of how to adapt – both mentally and physically. These changes disrupt our individual perceptions of our beauty, desirability, and value, while quietly giving us the opportunity to redefine and re-examine our beliefs about those things.

So, how do we strive for a new definition of beauty after experiencing hair loss?

HAIR CARE SPECTRUM

by Luciana Naldi

As I head into the menopause transition at 46 years old, I reflect back to the way I felt at the onset of my hair disorder. At that time, my appearance was already something I was self conscious of. I am Italian, and have an Italian (read: Large) nose, which was definitely the brunt of jokes growing up. In addition, I wasn't the Sophia Loren kind of Italian. I didn't have voluptuous curves or long hair, but my three sisters did and that was also pointed out. So adding hair loss when I already felt I was cheated genetically seemed like a cruel joke.

A dermatologist sat me down and said, "You have alopecia." I asked what that was and she said, "It's where your immune system attacks your hair follicles for reasons we don't know and don't understand, causing it to either come out everywhere on your body, or as in your case, in patches in a specific place. I see you still have hair on your eyebrows and some on your arms, so it doesn't look like you have the kind that is universal. I believe it's alopecia areata, which is characterized by round patches of hair falling out."

For a while, I was able to treat my alopecia with a first line treatment of Rogaine. My hair grew back, but as I entered my mid-thirties it fell out again, and this time nothing worked.

I went through what I now call a "hair care spectrum." For me, the hair care spectrum was the emotional spectrum I felt I was moving along throughout this process. It started with "I care," which meant: I do care about how I look, how my hair feels falling around my face and down my back, how beautiful my hair looks to me and others, how beautiful I feel with hair. This part of the spectrum lasted three or four months, during which time I also tried a majority of the "solutions" the doctors suggested for me – none of which worked. I think I would've stayed in this phase of the spectrum much much longer had I been single, had I not had children, or had I been in a profession more focused on my appearance. Having my own children literally watch me every day as I emotionally and physically dealt with this stripped away any and all cares about what I needed to be for anyone else except them, and what I wanted to be for myself. What and whose ideas about who I am did I really want to listen to? How could I communicate and embody with my actions the major values I was trying to instill in my children about body image, identity, and resilience? I would not have felt as much urgency to move along the spectrum without the curious and very raw questions of my children. I moved from *I care* to *can I not care* after visiting the doctor that asked me questions about what I valued and what I wanted to do.

Part of my process of moving along the hair care spectrum towards *indifference* was the deeply meaningful conversations I had with women who'd approach me and share their stories of hair loss, cancer, or physical hardship. They either offered their genuine support that I could get through what I was going through and be okay on the other side, or they expressed joy at seeing another woman moving through the world like they were.

The interaction that stands out the most to me was with a woman that had to be in her late seventies. I was sitting with my mom at a small bakery, which was rare, because I am hardly alone with my mom since having children. We were enjoying time visiting, cozied around some coffee when an impeccably dressed, petite older woman approached me with tear-filled eyes. She quietly came within whispering distance, paused and said, "You are so brave. I have wanted for years to do it and just could not. My husband wouldn't support it."

As she finished, her hand went to the hair right above her eyebrows and she slowly moved it back, revealing it was a wig and her own bald head underneath, before putting it back in place discreetly. Her tears fell silently as she patted me on the shoulder and walked away. The tears that came for me as she walked away were not because she had told me I was brave, because I didn't feel brave. Brave was reserved for people who did heroic things in times of great distress, or challenge. Existing as a bald woman because I wanted to was more rebellious than brave in my mind. My tears came because this woman had to appear to be someone else in order to survive in her own life, and I don't think anyone should have to do that. We aren't here to hide who we are.

Today, I am firmly on the indifference end of the spectrum – the end that can look at beautiful hair on other women and appreciate it. The one that knows that each person is going to have completely different opinions, ideas, and feelings about hair, beauty, their body, and how it all fits together and supports their right to do what feels best for them. I operate very much from the perspective of not judging other's choices when I don't know what their options are. When people come to me with questions or the need to share what they're experiencing in hopes of finding some kind of direction or anchor, I ask if it's advice they need or just an ear. Most people need and want a witness to their pain or sadness so they don't suffer alone, and that's okay with me. I had people hold my heart through all of this and I'm happy to hold the hearts of others if it helps.

WHERE TO TURN FOR HAIR LOSS HELP

Your primary care physician (PCP) is a great starting place to assess whether you have hair loss caused by an underlying condition, medication, supplements, hormone changes, or aging. They will typically send a letter summarizing the problem to a specialist. However, this was not my experience. I mentioned my hair loss to my OB/GYN and I remember asking her if this could be a problem with my thyroid. She replied, "It's probably not that." And that was the end of our conversation.

I never returned to that doctor, so I don't know if she simply didn't have time to assess what it might be, or if she didn't know the full details of this issue. What I do know is that menopausal women have been underserved. I mention this because it's important to go into medical appointments with questions. If you are not getting satisfactory answers, you need to request someone who has specialized expertise. You are a consumer of healthcare, and it's important to be a good advocate for yourself. This is called "collaborative decision making" and it's an important concept, because we have a very patriarchal model in medicine, e.g. my doctor tells me what to do and I do it.

Collaborative decision making means being aligned and partners with your doctor in supporting your health.

The specialist, in my case, was a board-certified dermatologist who specializes in hair loss treatment. They are well versed in the many options available to help regrow hair. A timely referral to specialty care is an important goal for all treatment options for FPHL, in order to prevent progression of hair loss rather than promote hair regrowth. The type of treatment your doctor prescribes will depend on the cause of hair loss.

YOUR BODY NEEDS ADEQUATE NUTRITION FOR HAIR GROWTH

When ruling out whether you are presenting with a hair disorder or other underlying causes, questions about diet will be at the forefront. As an eating disorder therapist, hair loss is something I often see in my caseload, and it can be the result of an energy imbalance that occurs when someone is not meeting their energy needs. This can happen intentionally, due to dieting, or unintentionally when someone is exercising a lot and fails to eat enough to meet their needs. Either way, the effect on the body is the same. There is not enough fuel to support non-essential functions such as hair growth; instead, the body prioritizes more essential functions such as keeping the person's heart beating and the brain working (though usually that gets a little foggy under these circumstances). When nutrition is inadequate, dead hair will eventually fall out, causing receding hairlines, diffuse hair loss, and/or dullness or a "lack of shine" to the hair. Alteration in hair can be so unsettling for our clients that is often a powerful motivator for recovery. Underfueling might not be the primary reason for hair loss, especially if the client is in the age range of natural menopause, but it can definitely enhance the problem.

Balancing Energy

Did you know that an energy imbalance, which is a mismatch of energy in vs. energy out, can affect hair loss? Those who are at risk for experiencing an energy imbalance include:

- Athletes or those who spend a lot of time exercising
- Individuals with limited food preferences

- Those with severe allergies
- Vegans, and anyone undergoing a major change in diet
- Those who lack interoceptive awareness (the ability to be aware of internal sensations in the body)
- Women taking medications that alter hunger/satiety cues
- Those experiencing food insecurity
- Anyone going through a major life transitions
- Anyone with a known eating disorder
- Those with mental health concerns such as depression, anxiety, or OCD, which may interfere with one's ability to self-nourish
- Those with GI concerns such as nausea, gastroparesis, bloating, constipation
- Any medical condition that alters appetite

If you are at risk for an energy imbalance or concerned with how to close the energy gap, a referral to a non-diet dietitian would be ideal to help you work on improving overall nutrition, including how to get back to incorporating regular meals and snacks. I also recommend the book *How to Nourish Yourself Through an Eating Disorder: Recovery for Adults Using the Plate-by-Plate Approach®* for those looking for guidance with eating disorder recovery.

UNDERSTANDING SKIN CHANGES WITH AGE

For those of you relating to my theme of coming of age in the 80s, products like "Sun In," baby oil mixed with iodine as "suntan lotion," and tanning stickers in the shape of Playboy bunnies (nod to Aunt Cindy) might sound familiar to you. But as my Gen Z daughter reminds me, "It's '*sunscreen*,' as in protection from the hydrogen broiler in the sky, not 'suntan lotion,' as in (the look on her face said,) 'What were you people thinking?'"

I explain to her that science might have tried to increase our awareness of the link between sun exposure and skin cancer, but our Gen X sensibilities dismissed science for a fashionable coconut-oil-basted bronzed exterior – and an unlit clove cigarette dangling from our fingertips (a story for another time)... According to The Menopause

Society, the face is the area of the body for which menopausal women seek the most medical advice. They note:

> Genetic makeup (intrinsic aging) combined with environmental and lifestyle choices (extrinsic aging) influence the clinical changes in the largest organ in one's body, the skin. As menopause approaches and estrogen levels fall, there is a resultant decrease in fibroblast activity (leads to a decrease in the regenerative abilities of the skin and the progression of aging), and less collagen is produced. The net effect is formation of lines and wrinkles and skin laxity.
>
> (Crandall, 2023, pp. 29-30)

Additionally, TMS suggests an annual skin examination by a dermatologist for patients with personal or family history of skin cancer.

A dermatologist is a medical doctor who specializes in the diagnosis and treatment of skin, hair and nail conditions. Based on the individual needs of each patient, they develop treatment plans that may include topical and oral medications, skin surgery on a specific area (such as to remove a growth,) observation, or a combination of these techniques. Additional patient-oriented information on skin-related topics can be found on the American Academy of Dermatology website (*American Academy of Dermatology*, 2025).

THE ART OF AGING

by Connie Sobczak

To age with grace and humor or to fight the inevitable physical changes that come with middle and old age – this is a choice we can make daily, if we are lucky enough to get to these life stages. Sadly, I know a lot of people who didn't make it to this stage, including my sister Stephanie, who died at age 36 because she hated her body.

When Stephanie died, I made a pact with myself to have as much fun as I possibly could for the rest of my days. It was a beautiful moment of insight in which I consciously realized that being mean to myself and letting my inner critical voice run the show was not my idea of fun! I've had many hard times since those days in my thirties, and yes, my critical voice has been something I've continued to work on, but as I've aged – I'm now 65 – I've always known how privileged I am to be getting old. My sister didn't have this opportunity, so in her name, I have made the choice to do the work every single day of liberating my body and growing in self-love.

Something that baffles me is how so many people become uptight and fearful about being "healthy" in order to live into old age, but when they get to the old age part, they hate their bodies because they are old! So they start in with cosmetic surgery and diets and whatever the latest fad is, and forget that it is a gift to become old.

I'm not saying it's easy. The skin changes that come with growing older present an interesting challenge. I see all body (including skin) changes as *challenges* rather than *problems*, which helps tremendously in allowing each one to be incorporated into my ever-changing and ever-expanding definition of beauty.

I read somewhere that when everyone started spending more time on Zoom because of COVID, a lot of people went to surgeons to "fix" their necks. They freaked out seeing the loose neck skin that is most definitely a part of the aging process. My response was, instead, to start really looking at my neck and honoring that it's old! I allow my eyes to fully take in the image I see of myself, of my skin changes on my neck and face. It's a powerful meditation process I undertake in these moments, and though it's not easy, over time it works.

I tell folks all the time how happy I am to be an old lady. As you can imagine, the first response from many is to say, "You're not old!" And my response is, "Yes, I *am* old. I'm in my third act, and if I'm lucky, I'll get older and older and my skin will become more wrinkled and saggy, and I'll be like the wise, beautiful crone that my precious mama was when she left the earth at the age of 96."

I had a beautiful, age-affirming experience recently, when I was about to take my grandson out for a walk. My daughter was applying sunscreen to both of our faces, his smooth as silk, and mine, rough and marked. As she was rubbing in the cream she said, "Oh, I love seeing your face getting older. It's so beautiful!" And I believed her.

Instead of saying, "Yuck, my skin is ugly, especially compared to your young skin," I simply said, "Thank you." I soaked in her words, which were her truth. My daughter sees my aging skin as beautiful, just as I saw the same in my own mama. I'm grateful for this family legacy of expanding our definition of beauty to include old skin, instead of passing on fear of our skin as we move through life.

I do use sunscreen now, as I don't want to get skin cancer. And growing up when I did, I have had more than enough sun exposure! But I still love the sun, and sometimes I forget to lather myself up or grab my hat when I'm out in my garden or going for a short walk, so chances are, I'll get more age spots on my arms and my hands will continue to turn into tree bark. And since I'm not planning to have cosmetic surgery (which is what killed my sister), I will allow my neck to become an old person's neck. I now see my neck skin as rings on a tree. And I absolutely love old trees!

I can't talk about aging with grace and humor without also mentioning my hair. I started getting gray hair when I was sixteen years old, and it really started going gray when I was in my late thirties. I inherited my wild, gray, curly hair from my mom. People think I'm making a political statement by having gray (now more white than gray!) hair. But for me, I simply think it suits who I am. I have lots of friends who dye their hair and it looks lovely. I'm not judgmental at all. It's just that I don't think I'd look good with a different color, and I've also grown into it over time.

I remember when my daughter was in elementary school, a boy asked me if I was Carmen's grandmother. I said, "No, I'm her mom, but I'm guessing you think I'm her grandma because of my hair." He concurred, and I gave him a simple, gentle lesson about how bodies are different and some people have this color hair before they are old. Around that same time, the UPS delivery person at my office, whom I had known in my twenties when my hair was jet black, said, "I hope you're not offended, but doesn't it bother you that when people see you from behind, they think you're old?" Again, a teaching moment to share how I feel about being my authentic self. My gray hair is definitely a signature part of my authenticity!

It takes courage to see our aging bodies as beautiful and valuable in a world that idealizes youthful appearance; a world where people and corporations make huge profits when we see our aging selves as ugly and unworthy. I will leave you with the practice that has helped me allow my precious self to move into old age with joy and grace: The way to redefine beauty and to continually include ourselves in the definition is by sitting in meditation with the parts of ourselves that we have been conditioned to become afraid of, until we are able to shift the way our eyes see and to then see these parts with loving kindness and acceptance. We keep at this practice (and I'm not saying it's easy!), allowing the subtle nuances of what beauty can be in an aging human body to come through over time.

Many changes will happen to your body as you grow older and move through menopause – it's something we can't avoid if we are lucky enough to live a long life. I'm glad you've found your way to this book, because you'll learn new and lasting ways to incorporate these changes into your life with as much ease and peace as possible.

REFERENCES

American Academy of Dermatology. (2025). https://www.aad.org/

Crandall, C. (2023). *Menopause practice: A clinician's guide* (6th ed.). North American Menopause Society.

Darpinian, S. (2023a, October 26). *Menopause, nutrition and diet culture: Getting the facts straight on midlife health*. Audioboom. https://audioboom.com/posts/8408208-menopause-nutrition-and-diet-culture-getting-the-facts-straight-on-midlife-health

Darpinian, S. (2023b, October 6). *The wonders of the changing female body-menopause, midlife and beyond*. Audioboom. https://audioboom.com/posts/8376690-the-wonders-of-the-changing-female-body-menopause-midlife-and-beyond

Godman, H. (2023, January 1). *It's not too late to save thinning hair*. Harvard Health. https://www.health.harvard.edu/diseases-and-conditions/its-not-too-late-to-save-thinning-hair

Schonberg, V. (2023, October 26). *The weight of menopause*. Midlife Health & Nutrition Solutions – Val Schonberg RD MSCP. https://valschonberg.com/the-weight-of-menopause/

PART 2

Cultivating Midlife Mental Health

Your Changing Emotions

Three

As women enter midlife and approach menopause, they can experience a unique set of internal and external vulnerabilities that impact their mood. As you saw in the preface, my mood symptoms while traversing menopause were somewhere in the "high middle." As I'm writing this book, I am realizing that we don't have a way to articulate symptom severity as it relates to hormonal fluctuation in this phase of life. In our reproductive years if we have mood symptoms related to hormonal changes during our cycle, we call it premenstrual syndrome (PMS), if the disturbance in mood is much more severe and debilitating we might be assessed for premenstrual dysphoric disorder (PMDD). After pregnancy, a sharp drop in estrogen and progesterone can lead to hormonal imbalances affecting mood, which is called postpartum depression (PPD). Understanding what is happening physiologically can help us normalize the experience and seek effective treatment.

Not everyone who traverses menopause will experience mood related symptoms, but being aware that there is risk will help individuals not feel so blindsided by emotional dysregulation if it does happen. Dr. Jen Gunter, author of *The Menopause Manifesto*, writes, "One of the strongest risk factors for depression in the menopause transition is a previous history of depression. This suggests that some women have a biological vulnerability to the interplay between hormonal changes and depression, as the existence of PMDD and postpartum depression suggests" (Gunter, 2024; Behrman & Crockett, 2024).

In my interview with Lou Ann Brizendine, neuropsychiatrist at the hormone clinic at UCSF, she noted there can be as high as a 14-fold increase in depression, irritability, and anxiety during the transition years (Darpinian, 2023; Schmidt et al., 2004). "It might not be the

DOI: 10.4324/9781003632245-5

same every day – it may not be continuous, but it really is a big mental change in your mood and happiness," says Brizendine. Brizendine starts by test-driving options with her patients, from hormones to antidepressants. I can relate to the PMS-like symptoms intermittently throughout the month, marked by hormone instability, with spikes and dips in mood. As a therapist who didn't receive any guidance about the transition from my OB/GYN, I didn't know who to turn to. This was exacerbated by the notion that if you are in a "helping profession" you are supposed to *have it all together*. In my interview with Suzannah Neufeld, LMFT, CEDS and author of *Awake at 3 AM: Yoga Therapy for Anxiety and Depression in Early Pregnancy and Early Motherhood*, she said, "Knowing the signs of depression and anxiety doesn't prevent them from happening. Use the knowledge to set up support for yourself, not to judge yourself" (Darpinian, 2022a).

Judgment, unfortunately, is part of many women's health journeys, specifically with menopause. I had a conversation at a social event with a contemporary. We spoke about how difficult my menopause had been, how I dealt with problematic symptoms with little medical support, and how I had to advocate for myself to start MHT.

She replied, "Menopause is natural, we shouldn't need to take anything for it. I only use 'natural' remedies." I felt immediately judged. My story was framed back as a moral shortcoming, when it was, in fact, a story about self-advocacy for my well-being about an undoubtedly natural process.

I spoke to a colleague and friend, Shelley Aggarwal, MD, MS, who is an allopathic physician who advocates for integrative healthcare. I discussed the situation with her and she said:

> Informed decision-making is everyone's right. At the heart of informed decision-making is rich and balanced information that allows people to choose integrative and allopathic and other treatment modalities that are aligned with their beliefs and preferences. Unfortunately, this was an undermining comment that identified "natural remedies" as the right choice and all other options as the wrong ones. As for something being qualified as natural and thus not being aided by advances in healthcare, think about the advances in contraception options and the ability to manage reproductive choice. Think about taking an over-the-counter pain reliever for a headache. There are many aspects of life that can

be placed under various labels of good and bad. However, this is rarely helpful. There is benefit from meaningful medical advances in every discipline, including integrative medicine disciplines, that can support health. And collaborative approaches may further support well-being. It doesn't have to be either/or, but it should always be as safe as possible. Let's not limit ourselves through the phenomenon of "othering," especially if it puts us at odds and prevents discussion.

Every treatment method should consider risks and benefits and all persons investing time, money, and other resources in various care options should ask thoughtful questions about how this treatment will serve them – and if it is safe. In my interview with Neufeld, she touched on how an "all natural mandate" can cause harm. Treatment for certain symptoms, specifically mood disruption, may be delayed. The bottom line is that neither supplements or medications are all good or all bad, and women deserve accurate, comprehensive information about both, so they can conduct their own risk-benefit assessment of what works for them.

This chapter is full of skills and tools you can use for mood disruption, stress, sleep disruptions, brain fog, bereavement, and more. These are themes we are bound to face in midlife and beyond. The bigger the array of interventions, the easier it will be to pick and choose what is right for you. The interactive prompts will help you integrate the material, as well as reduce emotionally aroused states. If you keep practicing these skills, you will become savvy at knowing what skill set you should use based on the current emotional state you're in. Most of the explorations are preceded by a sample to help you gain insight or to give you suggestions for how to go about them. Note that if you pick up the skills and tools in this chapter, in an attempt to reduce internal vulnerabilities, and you notice the skills are collapsing too quickly, it might be time to schedule an evaluation with a specialist to assess additional treatment options and strategies.

GETTING STARTED

Women are often in a role of caretaking others, sometimes at the expense of their own well-being. They can tend to be out of practice tuning into their own needs and giving a voice to the love and support they need. Add to this that it's hard to know where to turn for help, and even if you find help, it can take a while to be seen by the various providers you need. Below is an exercise adapted from *Awake at 3 A.M.:Yoga Therapy for Anxiety and Depression in Early Pregnancy and Early Motherhood* (Neufeld, 2018), designed to help you take stock of the ways you would like to be supported when you are feeling vulnerable and waiting for care. Says author Neufeld, "This is a good exercise to do when you find yourself in need of support but can't think of exactly what to ask for. Even if you are feeling balanced or well-supported, consider doing the exercise as a way of taking care of yourself ahead of time – so that if you are in need in the future, you don't have to think too hard and can draw on what you've done here."

PRACTICE HONESTY WITH FRIENDS AND FAMILY (NEUFELD, 2018)

Asking for support means remembering that people can't read our minds. Below are some ways to ask:

- Be patient with me if I need to do a reality check with you when I feel insecure about a social interaction – maybe remind me that my insecure thoughts are the anxiety talking.
- Please show me some grace during this vulnerable time. The menopause transition is long and comes in waves – some years. I'll be more social and other times, I'll need to go more inward, and I might decline a fun invitation to go out. Please trust my care for our relationship, and have faith that I am doing my best to show up as best as I can.
- Taking walks is a great way for me to get outside, take deep breaths, and feel good in my body. They are even better with a friend. It's also a good way to be social without draining my battery. If you have time available, schedule a time for us to go on a walk. Or even better, find a weekly or monthly time to walk together.
- Make it safe for me to tell you I'm not doing well. Please ask me how I'd like you to listen to me. I might just need to vent, or I might want advice. I will do the same for you.
- Remind me that none of us have it all together. Let me know if you are struggling with the menopause transition, too! I'll be here for you! It feels good to be in it together.

- Please be patient as I go through ups and downs. One month I may have trouble with sleep, another, I may be really thriving. Let's comfort each other through struggles and celebrate our wins together.
- If I say I need to take some obligations off my plate, please support me in that. You don't need to tell me I can do it all or that I'm strong. It's okay to let me be fragile sometimes, or to honor me needing to slow down. I hope we can make space to brainstorm ways to increase self-care and reduce striving.

The reasons for mood disruption in midlife and menopause are multifactorial. Hormonal shifts affect mental health, the physical symptoms we talked about in Chapter One aren't exactly mood enhancers, there's an increase in health problems in midlife, and we may experience the loss of loved ones or changes in career and marital status, empty nesting, sleep disruption, and more. Not to mention stressors of the "sandwich generation" (a nickname for the mostly female, mostly middle-aged group of Americans who serve as caregivers for both older and younger family members at once) (Lei et al., 2023). A client of mine told me she notices the difference in the way she's treated as she ages; people look at her now like she's frail and in need of assistance, when in reality she's quite strong.

Early perimenopause is associated more with irritability, and late perimenopause more with anxiety, depression, and VMS (Santoro, 2024). The menopause transition is considered by the menopause societies to be a "window of vulnerability" (Makeba, 2024). The experience can be radically different from one woman to the next – smooth for some and debilitating for others, so the more options we have at our disposal, the more individualized the care can be. As you saw in Chapter One, mood-related symptoms are the third most reported symptoms by women, the first being hot flashes/night sweats (VMS), and the second being disrupted sleep, both of which affect mood. In simpler terms, "not feeling like myself" is normal during this time, so much so that it even has its own acronym in the menopause space: NFLM. Seeking help depends on where you are on the continuum and how much you feel that your symptoms are affecting your quality of life. Women say that what often helps them is just knowing what it is – they just want to know what's happening and what to expect across time. To date, women have not been given the anticipatory guidance they need to understand what is happening to them as they enter the transition.

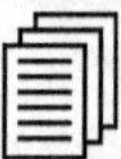

Exploration: Practice Honesty with Friends and Family

What are ways your loved ones can help you?

1.

2.

3.

4.

5.

When people find the courage to let their loved ones know they are struggling, and are able to educate them about the ways they can help, the feedback I hear from my client's support people is often, "Thank you for telling me how to be there for you."

As a therapist, I'm always assessing internal and external vulnerabilities that might be affecting clients' moods. For example, if someone has a pattern of under-eating, under-sleeping, and a sedentary lifestyle, it will be hard to assess things like mood symptoms, because these behaviors worsen mood. A client and I might work together to reduce external and internal vulnerabilities by making sure they are fueling adequately, working on reducing sleep disruptions, and getting in the habit of moving. Then we can develop a clearer picture of where their mood actually is. Food, sleep, and exercise should always have a seat at the table when discussing mental health.

WHAT IS COGNITIVE BEHAVIOR THERAPY?

Behavioral therapy in the early 20th century formed the first wave, and Beck's Cognitive Behavioral Therapy (CBT) the second. CBT was developed by Dr. Beck in the 1960s based on his research into the role of our thoughts and beliefs on our emotions. CBT is used to manage the thinking that gives rise to suffering. Since that time, when it was first discovered to be very effective in treating depression, it was exported for the use of other things, such as anxiety and the management of physical symptoms. In the menopause space, CBT is often used for the treatment of menopause symptoms such as hot flashes and night sweats, depression, anxiety, and sleep disruption (Makeba, 2024).

Over the last 30 years, the authors of *Managing Hot Flushes and Night Sweats: A Cognitive Behavioural Self-Help Guide to Menopause (Second Edition)* have developed CBT interventions specifically for menopausal symptoms based on years of research demonstrating the significant impact that psycho-social factors have on a woman's experience of menopause. The authors, Hunter and Smith, say, "The aim of CBT when applied to menopause is to help you identify unhelpful or overly negative beliefs and behaviors in relation to menopause and menopausal symptoms, to help you develop self-supportive and proactive management strategies" (Hunter & Smith, 2014, p. 49). Hunter and Smith write:

> Often and not surprisingly people tend to think that offering a 'psychological' treatment for a physical symptom means that the symptom is caused by the psychological factors. They fear that it's 'all in their head' or that they are 'going mad' in some way. We are brought up to view the mind and body as separate entities, but in fact health conditions affect us at all levels, and psychological, social and biological factors can influence our experiences of illnesses.
>
> (Hunter & Smith, 2014, p. 55)

A behavioral approach doesn't mean exclusion of hormone therapy or antidepressants, a combination of both (if needed) is considered the most effective, but not everyone is eligible to take HT, and it also doesn't work for everyone.

The word cognitive is fancy for "thoughts" or "thinking," and the "behavioral" part of the equation refers to "the observable actions and activities a person engages in." CBT puts an emphasis on secondary responses to primary emotions or physical states. For example, I might notice a warming sensation in my chest and face, and have a secondary response to that primary physical sensation.

> Oh my gosh, this room full of people can see my face turning red, and sweat dripping down my face. They are looking at me and wondering why I'm sweating so much. They're all going to know I'm having a hot flash.

That's an example of a secondary response to a primary physical sensation, which is likely to increase suffering and in turn exacerbate my hot flash.

A more balanced thought might be:

> I just noticed a warming sensation in my chest and on my face. I am having a hot flash. They tend to last 1–5 minutes, and this is just my brain's way of trying to regulate my body's temperature now that I have less estrogen. If someone notices it, fine, this is a natural symptom of menopause that half of the population will experience at some point. The more people that know about them the better. Hot flashes should be normalized.

This is an example of "cognitive reframing in an emotional state," a CBT skill that encourages us to look at a situation in a different way, ultimately decreasing emotionally aroused states. I like to make sure clients understand that these tools and skills aren't transformative, but instead they help a little bit more than not doing them. Sort of like the difference between a tablespoon of salt in a bucket of water versus the same amount in your Stanley.

Another CBT skill that's effective for cognitive reframing in an emotional state is called a Thought Record. When we are feeling out of balance due to hormonal fluctuations or life events, the brain has a tendency to fall back on our favorite negative stories, known as our "greatest hits." We all have them. You will notice that your life themes will get activated when your mood is disrupted, it's also known as "recall emotion." One way to know you are experiencing recall emotion is when you notice your feelings are bigger than the here and now. In these times you can ask yourself, "Is this recall or is this reality?"

The brain has a negativity bias even when we are not experiencing mood disruption, because its main feature is avoiding harm. This is a useful part of the brain that protects us and keeps us safe; without it, we might accept an invitation to get in a stranger's van full of puppies. However, we don't need the negativity bias to the extent that we have it now that we aren't living in caves, but the brain evolves very slowly. Dr. Rick Hanson, author of *Hardwiring Happiness*, says, "The brain is like velcro to negativity and teflon to positivity." We can let our brain use us, or we can choose to be more intentional and shift our perspective to more balanced thoughts. Below is a sample of a Thought Record. Writing these out can be highly useful when you're feeling distressed. Over time you'll find you can do them "imaginally" in your head for more run of the mill worries.

EXPLORATION: THOUGHT RECORD

Intensity of thoughts on a scale of 1-100%: 70%

Primary emotions (or physical symptoms): Anxiety, embarrassment, depression

Automatic thought (worse case scenario): At the pool today, everyone was talking in our group, but when I tried to chime in, it felt awkward. I'm too much, my personality is too big, they don't like me, I don't fit in. I feel anxious inside and everyone can tell.

Evidence to support automatic thought: Every time someone asked me a question and I started to answer, the person asking the question would get interrupted and they never came back to the question.

Evidence not to support automatic thought and a more balanced thought: I'm not feeling like myself (NFLM). I know that it's my hormones. I just have a couple of weeks until my appointment at the hormone clinic. Until then, I will do my best to not make my hormonal fluctuation my reality.

In my interview with Dr. Dan Tomasulo about his book *Learned Hopefulness*, he said, "It's not the one-off negative thought that's the problem, it's the rumination that's the real culprit" (Darpinian, 2022b). A Thought Record helps to stop the rumination that the mind tends to gravitate toward, which wanders far past the point of learning anything new and instead tends to further harm us.

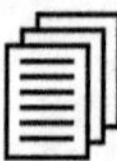

Exploration: Thought Record

Intensity of thoughts on a scale of 1-100%:

Primary emotions (or physical symptoms):

Automatic thought (worse case scenario):

Evidence to support automatic thought:

Evidence not to support automatic thought and a more balanced thought:

Lisa Mosconi, PhD, author of *The Menopause Brain*, states that postmenopause brings forth better emotional control related fine-tuning in the emotional amygdala. "With 50-plus years of life experience under their belts, many postmenopausal women have developed a nice set of skills, giving them a greater confidence they can handle whatever comes their way" (Mosconi, 2024, p. 98). I notice this myself, and observe this with the clients I support in my practice. Having a dysregulated mood in our late 40s and 50s is different than in our younger years; there's a self awareness that accompanies it. Years of life experience and personal growth can create more distance between our moods and ourselves. It's akin to the difference between "watching the movie of yourself" versus "being in the movie of you." This is called "observing self." What's valuable about having some distance is that it gives us more of a choice about how we want to respond to our private experiences or life events.

THIRD WAVE CBT THERAPIES

Over the last two decades "third wave" CBT therapies have evolved, as well. Dialectical Behavior Therapy (DBT) and Acceptance Commitment Therapy (ACT) are both offshoots of CBT but have their own specific approaches to address different types of mental health concerns. DBT is particularly designed for managing intense emotions, and ACT emphasises psychological flexibility versus rigidity, and the use of values to motivate behavior.

BEHAVIORAL CHAIN ANALYSIS

A tool I like to start with comes from Dialectical Behavior Therapy (DBT) and is called a Behavioral Chain Analysis (BCA). Therapy sessions can sometimes feel a bit fragmented, like a shaken-up snow globe. Creating a chain is a great way to anchor the content from the session, kind of like setting the snow globe down on a table and watching the snowflakes settle. This tool helps to understand the sequence of events and factors that lead to problematic patterns. Once I fill out the chain in session, the client and I try to identify the "target behavior," defined as the behavior that, if addressed, would create the most amount of change. Below is an example of how we might use this technique in session. The BCA is a great tool for cultivating curiosity about a situation, accessing the information you need, and moving on.

The idea here is to not regenerate the information past the point of learning something new.

Reduce Internal and External Vulnerabilities:

Slept 6 hours

No breakfast, late lunch (got too hungry)

Hormonal fluctuations led to anxiety

Two glasses of wine

Prompting Event:

Negative feedback from a colleague at work.

Thoughts/Feelings:

"I can be impulsive, why didn't I think that through?"

"My colleague really doesn't like me."

Feelings of inadequacy and shame.

Problem Behavior:

Regenerating the worry thought about what my colleague thinks of me, far past the point of learning anything new.

Consequences:

Heightened anxiety and dysregulated mood.

Target Behavior:

I will target the first chain by eating adequately and not drinking wine for now, to see if my sleep improves. I will also target the third chain to manage my thoughts and feelings so that I can reduce my suffering in situations like this. I will do a "thought record" next time to help me return to baseline more quickly.

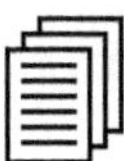

Exploration: Behavioral Chain Analysis

Reduce Internal and External Vulnerabilities:

Prompting Event:

Thoughts/Feelings:

Problem Behavior:

Consequences:

Target Behavior:

WHAT IF OUR EMOTIONS ARE INTENSE?

When emotions are more intense and the mind feels over engaged (churning at 100 percent), you might choose a skill that pulls you out of your current emotional state. This would likely stem from the distress tolerance module. Distress Tolerance is a DBT module meant for managing intense emotions. It's a skill that helps us put our pain up on a shelf temporarily and engage in an activity that helps reduce emotionally aroused states. The idea is to return to the pain once the emotion has eased a bit. Otherwise, overusing this module can lead to an accumulation of suppressed or blocked emotions.

Distress tolerance skills are a set of techniques designed to help us be able to hang out with uncomfortable emotions, without bringing in a behavior that makes the situation worse. This is also known as "bearing pain skillfully." For example, if every time a person experiences distress they use food as a way to cope, not only would the brain start to associate food with relief, but the chronic use of food in this way wouldn't lead to a diminishment of their original feelings. Feeding an emotion will only work while it's working – while we are eating the food – and it doesn't create a prolonged state of well-being. Once you are done eating, the emotion is right back up. Using food as the only way to cope would lead to suppression. (Note: Eating emotionally at times is a normal part of a peaceful relationship to food.) Many clients report that one of the ways chronic emotional eating serves them is that it grounds them. A DBT therapist might say that the bingeing is the client's solution, not the problem. The problem is difficulty hanging out in uncomfortable emotions without bringing in a behavior that makes the situation worse. If a person wanted to strengthen their ability to bear pain skilfully, and regulate emotions in ways other than turning to food, they could draw from a distress tolerance technique. When feeling an urge to binge, a great way to "act opposite" of the urge is to use a distress tolerance grounding technique.

EXPLORATION "54321"

5 things you can see: My lavender walls, my goldendoodle sleeping, logs in the fireplace, a magenta orchid, and my dirty breakfast plate.

4 things you can touch: My leggings, the blanket on my lap, the fleece in my sweatshirt, my furry dog.

3 things you can hear: An airplane overhead, my dog breathing while sleeping, people talking while walking by the front of the house.

2 things you can smell: The laundry soap on my sweatshirt, my dog's damp fur.

1 thing you can taste: My toothpaste.

Observing your environment in this way can gently bring you back into the present moment. It's a skill you can take with you anywhere, I'd suggest that you begin by practicing it when you are not in distress. The key here is fostering a more prolonged state of well-being that lasts well beyond the exercise.

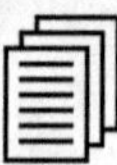

Now you try: Exploration "54321"

5 things you can see:

4 things you can touch:

3 things you can hear:

2 things you can smell:

1 thing you can taste:

THREE STATES OF MIND

The notion of Three States of Mind is a therapeutic tool that helps individuals understand and navigate the various ways in which their minds can operate, ultimately aiming to cultivate the Wise Mind, which balances emotion and reason. Imagine a Venn diagram with overlapping circles labeled Emotion Mind, Wise Mind, and Reasonable Mind. When we are thinking or analyzing, or using our intuition and feeling, we each tend to favor one of these states over the other. The goal is the integration of the two. With practice, you'll find it's empowering to know how to identify what state of mind you are in at any given time. Understanding the Three States of Mind provides an opportunity to press the pause button before taking action from an unbalanced place.

The first state of mind is called Emotion Mind. Signs that you're in "emotion mind" are black and white thinking, high emotion arousal, the feeling that *everything* is the truth, and often a driven or compulsive feeling in this state of mind. If at a given time one's primary emotion is anxiety, it's hard to know whether or not how we feel is "the anxiety talking." We can have a tendency to tweak the facts to match our feelings in this state. If it feels like someone's intention is malicious in this state of mind, then to our Emotion Mind, they are inherently malicious. Feelings become facts, and typically our feelings are bigger than the here and now. In perimenopause this is a state many women find themselves in sporadically.

Emotions are important, but in this state they are too high and they tend to edge out our more logical mind. In Emotion Mind, our amygdala – the part of the brain known for processing emotions such as fear, anxiety, and aggression – is activated. When this part of the brain is overly active, the prefrontal cortex – the part of the brain responsible for executive functions such as decision-making, cognitive control, and reasoning – is in a more dormant state. It's best to not take action out of Emotion Mind; instead, the goal is to identify this state of mind and engage in activities, such as the Distress Tolerance module, to pull yourself out of this heightened emotional state. Better to assess the reality of a situation when emotions return to baseline; otherwise, it's easy to take things overly personally.

Reasonable Mind is one of logic and reason. Think Spock from Star Trek. Reason and logic are obviously useful, but are best when integrated with our emotions and intuition. Otherwise there's a tendency to problem-solve with a sense of detachment from values and emotions. Operating solely from a Reasonable Mind might engender a lack of empathy and compassion, affecting interpersonal relationship skills.

Finally, there's Wise Mind. This is our sweet spot. Wise Mind is where you've arrived through the integration of Emotion Mind and Reasonable Mind, reflecting a "deepening," or confident sense of knowing. Here's an illustration. Imagine that a friend is dating someone new and tells you, "I desperately want to reach out to so-and-so right away…"

You can tell their desire has a driven quality to it, and you might advise them to wait until the feeling behind wanting to call has a more peaceful quality to it, something along the lines of, "I don't *need* to call, but I'd like to." That's Wise Mind in action – clear thinking and clarity of mind. Action taken in Wise Mind is referred to as taking "inspired action."

When developing your Wise Mind, pause and tune into yourself to identify what state you are in throughout the day. If you find yourself in Emotion Mind as evidenced by a feeling of anxiety, you might reach out to someone you trust who can help pull you back into Wise Mind, or at least support you in taking a pause before taking action in that state.

In a therapy session, a client of mine told me about an incident the prior week with her son. She said he was supposed to be helping her clean the house, which he had promised to do after spending all day with friends. In the middle of his designated chore time, she noticed he was "chilling" on his phone. She could feel her emotions rising as she said, "The house is a disaster, and you're clearly not helping!"

Her son snapped back, "I'm not done, I'm still cleaning!"

Not accustomed to him being reactive, she retreated to her room and started to tidy her dresser-top. This helped her to "act opposite" of her urge to yell back – or at least to press pause (something we had been working on together in therapy). Cleaning in her room helped put her emotions on the "metaphorical shelf" to de-escalate. Once her intense emotions eased and she was no longer engaging in black and white thinking ("You don't care about helping me, you just want to be on your phone,") she was able to access her Wise Mind, which told her something more was going on with her son.

She went back to her son's bedroom, lightly knocked on the door, and asked if she could come in. He felt remorse about yelling (she did, too), and they were able to talk about what was happening beneath the incident. My client was able to take responsibility for the stress she was under. The thing causing her stress was cleaning – something she, not her son, chose for him to do the minute he walked in the door. She told him she could do better, and said, "In the future I will ask you *when* you plan to do your chores."

Once she talked about her own stress about their untidy house, her son had the space to tell her that kids at school had been teasing him about having a female friend. He said that that day some kids were making kissing noises when he walked by with his friend. He asked, "Can't I just have a female friend without it becoming 'a thing?'"

It was a growth moment for both.

This anecdote from my client's home life is an example of initially being in Emotion Mind, pressing the pause button and engaging in a behavior to bring the emotion down, guaranteeing a quick return to baseline. Understanding the Three States of Mind offered her/my client an opportunity to assess which state she was in, and adjust accordingly.

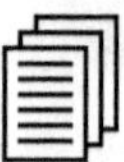

Exploration: Three States of Mind

Which state of mind do you default to, or spend the most time in?

Describe a time recently when you were in Emotion Mind. (Example: I can't stand waiting three days for so-and-so to call me after our first date. I have to call now!)

Describe a time recently that you were in Reasonable Mind. (Example: It's good to wait exactly three days before calling someone after a first date; it gives us both a chance to reflect on the experience and on each other. I will wait until tomorrow, because that will be 72 hours.)

Describe a time recently that you were in Wise Mind. (Example: It's been a couple days since my first date with so and so. Before worrying "did they like me," I did my own work and considered if I wanted to see them again; as it happens, I feel fine either way!)

ACCEPTANCE COMMITMENT THERAPY

When I was at my first Acceptance Commitment Therapy (ACT) training, I learned about the emphasis that theoretical orientation put on identifying values and adjusting behaviors to better match them. I had to raise my hand at this training and ask, "How are you defining values?" Of course I know what values are, but I needed to understand them in this context.

The workshop leader cited Russ Harris, author of *The Happiness Trap* (who popularized ACT): "Values are your heart's deepest desires for how you want to behave as a human being." They proceeded to show the attendees a list of sixty values from *The Happiness Trap*'s free resource list (Harris, 2010). Start by identifying your top values. What matters to you? What sort of person do you want to be at this stage in your life? Use those values to guide, inspire, and motivate you to take action toward your values.

One of the hallmarks of ACT is to think about and reconsider decisions that are controlled by negative emotions, as opposed to our core values. The goal is to put our values, not our negative emotions, in the driver's seat. In the ACT training, participants were given an example of a woman in recovery from her eating disorder feeling fearful of attending her niece's birthday party, because she felt anxiety around celebration foods such as cake. One of her core values was "family;" skipping the party would be acting in opposition to this value. Attending the birthday party is an example of taking valued action – taking action toward her value of family – whereas eating cake is an example of taking action toward her recovery.

The woman in this workshop example practiced "teaching her anxiety a lesson," by not allowing her anxiety to see and act. Avoiding "forbidden foods" might reduce her distress in the moment, but this behavior also keeps this woman from living a better life. In ACT this is called an "adaptive peak." Instead, she took an action-precedes-motivation approach; in other words, she didn't wait to get in the "mood" to go to the party, she just went to the party. She ate a piece of cake, which gave her an opportunity to realize that her fear was unfounded. Going to the party and having cake left her with a sense of self-mastery and self-trust. Going to the party *and* eating cake is the way she wants to show up for herself and others in her life. ACT in action!

BRINGING SEXY BACK

by Maeve

Maeve's core values: Compassion, honesty, humor, and love

Following divorce after a 19-year-marriage and two years of rebuilding my finances (and spirit!) as a single parent, I am dating someone new for the first time in more than two decades. I discovered quickly that I am as self-conscious about my body as I was in my twenties – perhaps moreso, since I've given birth to three children and gained additional weight in midlife. My ex-husband never, ever complimented me on my appearance or style and rarely touched me with affection. Over time, I stopped seeing myself as a sexual being entirely.

As I embarked upon a new monogamous relationship, I found I am shy about nudity when having sex or being intimate, and struggle to love my undressed body. My boyfriend noticed that I often cover my stomach, even when relaxing. He has even joked about how quickly I rush to throw on a t-shirt following sex, so that I spend as little time naked as possible. I want to enjoy my life and this relationship and not lose however-many-more years to self-judgment and self-doubt. Admittedly, that goal feels…Herculean.

My lifelong feelings of self-criticism and body shame, including daily thoughts about wishing I had a smaller body, hung over each interaction like a storm cloud, overriding the values I try to carry through the world and share with others – compassion, honesty, humor, and love. Where are my self-compassion and self-love? How can I be a feminist and judge my appearance with such hatred? Why do I subject myself to a harsh and punishing inner monologue that I'd never inflict on a friend or loved one? Am I risking ruining this happy and special time with a new partner because I can't accept my body and see myself as beautiful and deserving of love and sex?

Although the nature of my challenge – being comfortable naked – may seem minor in the grand scheme of life, for me it became all-consuming. My anxiety around undressing and my overall body-shyness weren't cute or quirky. They were a problem – a betrayal of my deep-held values – that I knew I had to address, and the sooner, the better.

After my first few lovely, romantic but admittedly awkward and (if I'm being honest) somewhat prudish encounters with my partner, I decided to tackle my shame head-on. One thing holding me back was sartorial – I was still wearing the worn-out undies and ill-fitting bras I'd defaulted to in, oh, the last ten or so years of my marriage. I drove to the mall and gritted my teeth while asking an adorable young saleswoman to help me determine my bra size. (*Good news! It was much less cringey than I'd feared!*) Armed with this new information, I treated myself to some quality lingerie, and my partner also delighted in surprising me with an avalanche of options once I shared my requested sizes with him.

Beautiful silks and satins *did* boost my confidence, but I also felt to an extent that I was simply dressing up my "flawed" figure. I knew I had to "teach my anxiety a lesson." As the daughter of a therapist, I've heard one line many times over in my life: "Fake it 'til you make it." This useful little phrase can apply to professional confidence, personal relationships, activities such as public speaking, performing or athletics competitions, and so much more. And now… nookie?

Here's where ACT therapy rode in on its white horse.

Here's where ACT therapy rode in on its white horse. I knew that to get over my initial fears, I needed to kick my negative feelings aside and act first…allowing the rest (genuine confidence and self-acceptance) to grow and blossom over time. And so, for the first time in my life, I acted confident and sexy! Me! I would strut into the room in a bodysuit or corset and strike poses for my partner. I performed a flirtatious fashion show of my new purchases. I admired myself at home, in the mirror, in bras and slips I'd never indulged in as a younger woman because *I didn't deserve them.*

I must acknowledge external factors as well – not just the beautiful new lingerie, but my partner's words and actions. He tells me I am beautiful multiple times a day, calls me a litany of pet names, and absolutely loves my body. When I say something self-critical or deprecating, he calls me on it. He has asked me directly not to devalue myself, something I struggle to ask of myself. I'd be lying if I said this didn't help enormously, and honesty is one of my core values! But I also know that we can't rely on others for our own self-worth, and so my path toward loving and respecting my body winds on.

I genuinely believe this journey will never end for me. Forty-five years of crushing cultural and media messages about beauty standards, years of childhood bullying, and marriage to a man who often proudly proclaimed, "I didn't marry you for your looks" (WTF!) have done a lot of damage and those scars remain. My current relationship may end one day, and if I find myself back in the dating pool, I will once again wonder how my appearance "measures up."

I continue to ask myself values-clarifying questions. How would I speak to a dear friend experiencing this in their own new relationship? What if I *am* beautiful and deserving of pretty clothes and frequent compliments? Is there another way to exist, now that I'm in midlife, in which I think of myself in loving and positive terms?

Surprising myself completely, I'm learning that confidence is sexy. I'm "faking" my feelings less and leaning into the joy of dressing up and seeing myself as a sexual creature again – or perhaps, truly, for the first time. Sometimes I throw on a sundress to grocery shop and clock appreciative glances from strangers in the aisles. I regularly use my limited discretionary money for things that make me feel beautiful – manicures, colorful socks, yoga workshops, short-ish dresses. I can be a feminist and embrace my own femininity; I wasted far too much time considering these things mutually exclusive. I can be a cheerleader and friend for myself, not just for others. I can be in a partnership that is respectful and body positive *and* feral and unabashedly sexual. And last – but not least – I can twirl around in a pink lace chemise without bursting into flames!

WHAT SKILL SHOULD I USE?

It might seem obvious, but the skill or tool you pick up really depends on your current emotional state. This chapter is about curating your toolbox; whether or not you are experiencing the intense emotions that can occur sporadically during the menopause transition, including sleep disruption, physical symptoms such as hot flashes, or run of the mill worry thoughts. Thought Records are very useful when you find yourself worrying beyond the point of learning something new. Identifying what state of mind you are in can help to create space between you and an impulsive action. The 54321 activity can help bring you into the current moment when your emotions are running wild.

SLEEPLESS IN PERIMENOPAUSE

I watched a master class with Dr. Matthew Walker, author of *Why We Sleep*, and I remember him saying, "Sleep is a time of reception, not reflection." I agree with Dr. Walker, but I don't think the dude has lived through perimenopause. What I would have given to know ahead of time that waking up at 3 a.m. was related to my menopause transition. I remember being so worried that sleepless nights were going to be the norm for me in midlife and beyond; I had no idea my sleeplessness was related to drops in my estrogen levels and night sweats, among other things. Some preliminary advice would have been amazing, because knowing that my experiences were common (and usually temporary) would have made everything feel easier and less existential! Sleep disruption and sleep disorders are a problem faced by teenagers and adults of all ages, but can be particularly egregious and miserable during women's midlife.

Ashley Brauer, Licensed Clinical and Sport Psychologist (PhD), and Diplomate in Behavioral Sleep Medicine (DBSM) says, "Sleep and health are intertwined, but sleep is often under addressed in the context of health problems." Sleep has a lot in common with menopause and women's health in that regard. Perimenopausal and postmenopausal women report significantly more sleep issues than premenopausal women. Adds Brauer, "Sleep is a core foundation of health. Sleep problems can exacerbate current health difficulties or contribute to the onset of new ones, and mental health difficulties will often exacerbate sleep problems. We can't talk about one without talking about the other."

MY LONG JOURNEY WITH INSOMNIA

by Alexsia

My insomnia began in my early to mid-30s after a stressful move across the country and then a hard break-up. I was not eating well, drinking too much caffeine, and was generally stressed out! I had also gone back to college after a long hiatus, so my brain was working overtime. I started waking in the middle of the night with repetitive thoughts and often with my pillow and sheets sweaty. This was strange and new. When I mentioned it to a holistic health practitioner, he suggested I may be in perimenopause (a term I was unfamiliar with at the time). I now know such early signs of perimeno-like symptoms can occur for a number of reasons.

My insomnia resulted in fairly constant brain fog as I was plagued by repetitive thought patterns that would keep me up in the middle of the night. I was looking for remedies all over the place and tried acupuncture, herbal medicine, and various supplements, all of which did give some relief for a limited amount of time. The night sweats did go away at this time.

At 38, I became pregnant and after the initial progesterone wash of the first trimester, the insomnia returned. Once I had my baby, I felt like the insomnia I experienced was way beyond what any other friends had described with childbirth (especially because it lasted for years). Every day I felt like the walking dead. At night, or when I'd try to have a nap, I would lay in bed worrying that not sleeping would make the next day so difficult to attend to any of my tasks with any sense of quality or pride. My brain fog and irritability was off the charts. My energy for parenting was so low and I felt guilty about that. My libido was down to zero too. I did not feel like myself – I didn't even really know myself anymore – and this went on for years.

During this period I tried sleep medication (Ambien) and I hated the way it made me feel. Though I was unconscious at night, I would wake feeling like I'd never gone to sleep. Melatonin made me feel sleepy and I would sleep, but, I'd wake super groggy every time I used it. What was the point of using these medications and supplements if I could sleep but then wake feeling totally unrested?

Finally, in my mid-to-late 40s, the insomnia subsided. It was still there, coming in waves (related to my menstrual cycle), but I had some tools in my toolkit now. I used meditation or listening to boring books or podcasts to lull me back to sleep. I was functional until true perimenopause hit (50-ish) and then I was struggling with insomnia again, along with the recurrence of hot flashes. Feeling very little patience for continuing to experiment with methods. I asked my doctor about hormone therapy and once I started my sleep improved. I finally felt like me!!

It's been amazing to feel "all the way alive." I've had a year of sleeping well and I love it. Over the past month, I have felt the insomnia creeping back in from external stressors, pain in my body, and caffeine later in the day, but it's only two to three times a week in contrast to the five days a week I used to experience. It's too early to tell, but if it does return, my plan is to use CBT-I, something I'm learning about now after 20 years of insomnia!

WHAT'S THE DEAL WITH SLEEP PROBLEMS IN MENOPAUSE?

by Dr. Ashley Brauer

Some version of Alexsia's story may sound familiar to you or someone in your life. As many as 70 percent of midlife women will complain of "sleep disturbance." The highest rate is in late perimenopause, as well as in women who have undergone surgical menopause (independent of chronological age) (Makeba, 2024). Sleep disturbance associated with menopause is different from other times in life due to the complex combination of numerous physiological changes and potential life stressors. This is an unfortunate reality for many and often does not receive the attention it deserves. It is common for society to write off sleep problems as "normal," or "just something you have to deal with."

The relationship between sleep disorders and other mental health concerns are bi-directional. The word "insomnia" is frequently used in casual conversation in today's society. The reality is that insomnia can mean different things, and this can create confusion, even among providers. Insomnia can be a symptom of another problem or develop into a disorder itself (what we call "insomnia disorder"). Alexsia's story demonstrates a classic pathway to the onset of insomnia – lots of stress, transition, and changes to diet and caffeine intake. In cases like Alexsia's, insomnia may start out as a symptom of physical or psychological changes, then develop into insomnia disorder, in which someone has trouble falling asleep, staying asleep, or waking up too early several nights a week for a significant period of time (typically longer than one month).

HOW DO SLEEP PROBLEMS DEVELOP?

There are many reasons why individuals experience sleep disruptions throughout perimenopause and menopause. First, we all have a unique set of genetic, personality, and health factors that may make us prone to developing insomnia. Being assigned female at birth is a vulnerability, as women are twice as likely to develop insomnia as men (Zhang & Wing, 2006). Second, something often triggers initial sleep problems. Examples include being awoken by night sweats or trouble falling asleep due to life stress. Sometimes it can be hard to pinpoint an initial event because hormonal changes (declining estrogen and progesterone) can contribute to difficulties falling asleep or waking up at night – in which case these hormonal changes may be the initial event that causes sleep difficulties. Sleep problems may improve once the initial trigger is resolved or treated. This is an example of insomnia functioning as a symptom, for example when an individual experiences a stressful event and notices short-term sleep disruption that goes away once the stressful event is over. Another example is if someone experiences sleep difficulties as a result of moderate or severe night sweats, and the sleep problems resolve with the hormone therapy that mitigates the night sweats. In Alexsia's case, the HT did provide minimal improvements to her sleep, but it could be observed that Alexsia had a predisposition and history of chronic sleep issues that likely represent insomnia disorder, so it would not be surprising that her insomnia is "creeping back in." She may greatly benefit from addressing sleep thoughts, feelings, and behaviors through Cognitive Behavioral Therapy Insomnia (CBT-I).

Finally, thoughts and behaviors can start to change around sleep. Have you ever gotten into bed earlier to try and sleep more? Or slept in to get more sleep? Perhaps you've noticed increased worry about lack of sleep? Or you're placing greater pressure on yourself to make sleep happen because you know how important it is? When thoughts and behaviors change around sleep, we might notice ongoing or worsening sleep problems. This is how insomnia becomes an ongoing problem and may develop into insomnia disorder. Alexsia continued to struggle on and off with sleep, to the point where sleep issues became a chronic problem in which her thoughts and behaviors started changing around sleep (e.g., "I would lay in bed worrying that not sleeping would make the next day so difficult to attend to any of my tasks with any sense of quality or pride.")

Understanding these three components of sleep problems is known as the "3P Model of Insomnia," which stands for Predisposing, Precipitating, and Perpetuating (Krystal et al., 2019). In Alexsia's case the Predisposing factor includes her vulnerability to chronic sleep issues, the Precipitating is the onset of perimenopause, and the Perpetuating factors include changing thoughts and behaviors around sleep (e.g., worrying in bed, belief that lack of sleep will diminish ability to do tasks the next day). The 3P model of insomnia is the foundation of the most well-studied treatment of insomnia, CBT-I, discussed in the next section.

COGNITIVE BEHAVIORAL THERAPY FOR INSOMNIA

The first line treatment, even before medication, is CBT-I. CBT-I is a structured, short-term, evidence-based treatment that specifically targets thoughts and behaviors around sleep that contribute to insomnia. CBT-I lasts approximately six to eight sessions. It is important to note that the number of treatment sessions may vary depending on the individual's unique needs. CBT-I can be helpful for people regardless of if they are experiencing insomnia as a symptom or disorder. In fact, a trained provider can help an individual determine, along with their medical treatment team, what role sleep may be playing in their situation.

An example of a CBT-I exercise we might use is called Constructive Worry at Bedtime. This is a CBT-I exercise assigned if getting out of bed isn't enough to interrupt nighttime worries. Getting out of bed is a common CBT-I intervention as well, because people start to associate bed with worry, and ideally bedtime is a time of "reception, not reflection."

The next step is "constructive worry." Constructive Worry is a method of managing the bedtime worry that's common when we no longer have the business of the day to distract us from our worries, and instead the stillness of the evening is conducive to worry. The exploration below is an adapted excerpt from the book *Overcoming Insomnia: A Cognitive-Behavioral Therapy Approach (Second Edition)* (Edinger & Carney, 2015). The authors suggest doing the exploration in the late afternoon or early evening (ideally two hours before bed). Fifteen minutes is the time typically allotted for this exercise (see Table 3.1).

Table 3.1 Sample Constructive Worry at Bedtime

Concerns	*Solutions*
Money is tight, I should start looking for another job.	There have been times before when money was tight and it's only been temporary. I will use this time to watch webinars, do my reading, and prepare for upcoming talks.
My son didn't get the part he auditioned for in the play.	This is a part of life. I will do my best to not short circuit the pain he's feeling and just allow him to process. I will tell him I'm here for him if he needs support.
I think I irritated my friend today by not agreeing with a stance she was taking on teenagers and social media.	It's okay to have differences of opinion, there are likely truths in what both of us are saying. I will sleep on it and decide tomorrow if I should revisit the conversation with my friend.

EXPLORATION: CONSTRUCTIVE WORRY AT BEDTIME

1. Write down the problems facing you that have the greatest chance of keeping you awake at bedtime, and list them in the "Concerns" column or in your journal.
2. Then, think of *the next step, or steps,* you might take to address each of the concerns you have listed. Write those down in the "Solutions" column. Remember that you don't need to have the final solution to the problem, since most problems are solved by taking a series of steps.
3. Repeat this strategy for all the concerns you may have.
4. After you do this exercise, close your journal (or this book), put it next to your bed, and forget about it until bedtime.
5. If at bedtime you begin to worry, tell yourself that you have dealt with your problems already in the best way you know how, and when you were at your best problem solving.
6. An additional benefit of the Constructive Worry technique may be less anxiety during the daytime.

BEYOND INSOMNIA

It's important to note that other sleep problems may present during perimenopause and menopause, so we shouldn't only limit our view to insomnia. It's important to assess for sleep apnea (partial or full disruption of breathing during sleep), snoring, nightmares, restless leg symptoms, and circadian rhythm disorders if sleep problems continue to persist. A great first step would be to contact your primary doctor and state, "I have been having problems with sleep and I am wondering if I could have a sleep disorder assessment. Could you help me with a referral to a sleep medicine clinic for a sleep study?" From there, sleep medicine providers will be able to complete an assessment and help you determine next steps for evaluation and treatment. To find a DBSM provider access the directory of Cognitive Behavioral Therapy Insomnia (CBT-I) providers (CBT-I *International Directory*, 2025).

SLEEP TIPS

You may have heard of the term "sleep hygiene." Sleep hygiene is a basic set of sleep habits that promote healthy and consistent sleep. Sleep hygiene is like brushing your teeth. It can help prevent problems and promote sleep health, but is not a treatment for insomnia or other sleep disorders, just as brushing your teeth is not the course of treatment for a cavity.

We can all benefit from establishing healthy sleep routines, just like we all benefit from brushing our teeth. I encourage individuals to pick one or two items on the list to work on at a time. Keep it simple and set yourself up for success.

Sleep Hygiene Tips

- Wake up at the same time each morning. This establishes our circadian rhythm, also known as our "body's clock". It is driven by a part of our brain called the suprachiasmatic nucleus, which operates like the body's orchestra conductor. Our body's clock is influenced by physical, mental, and behavioral changes. Aim to wake up at the same time on weekdays and weekends.
- Create a simple wind-down routine (e.g., phone away, brush teeth, read).
- Limit caffeine to earlier in the day. Aim to stop drinking caffeine at least six to eight hours before bedtime.
- Keep your bedroom dark, cool, and quiet.
- Use stress management before bed (e.g., breathing, stretching, time in nature).
- Avoid stimulating content before bed.
- Avoid napping or try to nap earlier in the day.
- Eat a snack before bed if you feel hungry. Note: You might see advice to not eat before bed, but listen to your body and decide what feels right to you. The last thing we want to be doing is fighting hunger at 3 a.m.!
- People often struggle to fall asleep soon after working out due to increased heart rate, body temperature, and increased physical stress. Listen to your body and decide if you need to move your workouts earlier in the day or give yourself more time to cool down before bed.
- Alcohol prior to sleep may make you feel sleepy, but will metabolize during sleep and can cause diminished sleep quality. Aim to reduce alcohol intake or stop consuming a minimum of four hours before bedtime.

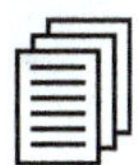

- Each person's circadian rhythm is different. Some are naturally "morning types" (known as larks) and some are "evening types" (known as owls). Our body clock can change as we age. Each person has a biological preference for their circadian rhythm.
- The public health recommendation for sleep for women in midlife is seven to nine hours, but there is appropriate variability outside of this window. It also likely depends on a variety of other factors, such as how much activity you are doing or overall health. There is no cookie cutter answer. The seven to nine hour recommendation is a good place to start, and individual sleep needs should be considered on a case-by-case basis.

BRAIN FOG

Rachel came back to me for therapy in her late fifties. The work we did previously was around her eating difficulties, but this time she was distressed about her symptoms of brain fog.

She noted that her sharp-as-a-tack persona was being tested by her memory loss and forgetfulness at work. Being detail-oriented and reliable was a big part of her identity, so this was very concerning to her. She was convinced she had early onset dementia. Rachel had a hysterectomy at age 44, and had not experienced any of the common physical manifestations of menopause, such as hot flashes, which made it difficult to know where she was in the menopause transition. In addition, she had difficulty sleeping, which can contribute to brain fog.

"I just made another major error at work. I'm feeling so demoralized. I have made enough errors in the last six months that my boss could fire me and it would be warranted," she shared in one session. "I don't think he will – assuming I can turn this around – but he is pretty pissed and with good reason. He has had to spend a lot of money fixing my errors. I'm equally stressed about getting fired and about my inability to function at a high level of accuracy that used to be second nature for me. Just this morning I made another error regarding our manufacturing schedule, but fortunately a colleague caught it before it was executed. It's another thing to add to the list of errors that I would have never made in the past."

40 to 60 percent of midlife women report cognitive symptoms such as forgetfulness during the transition. These symptoms manifest as brain fog, which reflects difficulty remembering words, names, anecdotes, and numbers; an inability to focus and concentrate; and distractibility (Maki & Jaff, 2022). Dr. Moscani, says, "Although *brain fog* is not a medical term, it aptly describes the fogginess in one's thinking, the mental fuzziness, and the difficulty processing information that often accompany menopause" (Mosconi, 2024, p. 49). Although it's common to fear early onset dementia when brain fog appears, in fact, only 293.1 women per 100,000 women worldwide develop early onset dementia (Maki & Jaff, 2024). Moscani says, "For context, dementia isn't forgetting where you left your keys. Dementia is forgetting what keys are for" (Mosconi, 2024, p. 54). There is robust evidence that typically brain fog reflects a temporary change, and that mental acuity recuperates after menopause.

Regular exercise and maintaining an extensive social network benefit memory and protect against dementia in the long run. You'll see more on improving these health behaviors in chapters to come. As we saw in Chapter One, hormone replacement therapy (HRT) is currently recommended for maintaining brain health only in women who have both of their ovaries removed (bilateral oophorectomy) before the typical age of menopause, or for those with premature menopause.

According to Moscani, if you are three to four years postmenopausal and you are still having serious concerns about your brain fog, and it is impacting your quality of life, it may be time to get tested by a neurologist or a neuropsychologist. In Rachel's case, she discovered that her brain fog might have been exacerbated by an undiagnosed sleep disorder, so her primary care physician started with a sleep test referral.

BEREAVEMENT IN MIDLIFE

Without question, of all the experiences we may have during midlife, one of the greatest potential stressors and sources of grief is the loss of a relative, partner or close friend. Losing a parent in midlife is a reality most of us are aware of but don't want to think about. This avoidance is compounded by the fact that we live in a grief-illiterate culture. Grief expert Dr. Linda Shanti notes, "Like most people, I had no experience with grief and death until grief and death happened to me" (Darpinian, 2024).

MEMORIES OF MOM

by Margaret Hunter, Licensed Marriage and Family Therapist (LMFT) and Registered Art Therapist (ATR)

I measure the time that has passed since my mother's death by the number of seasons that I have spent without her. Hot days of summer remind me of the joy I experienced with my mom. Long days at the beach; laughter in the sun; evenings spent reading and talking and dreaming about the future. The mystery and magic of springtime and the awakening of new life produces memories of the beautiful poetry she wrote. The poems described everything she observed in the world around her. I stroll through newly fallen leaves while taking in the smells of fall and winter, I remember her love of all seasons. I become painfully aware of all that I have lost since she has been gone.

During my daily mindful walks, I think of the road we traveled together and how my own life was profoundly affected by her life and her death. Even though my mother and I spent 60 years making memories together, it is the final years of her life that I remember the most. I associate winter with the beginning of our final journey together.

The dark winter season of my mother's life took place many years before her death. During this period a sadness crept in, as if delivered by a gentle storm looming in the distance. Mom had been living with crippling rheumatoid arthritis for many years. She adapted to the significant changes in her body, but she realized she would eventually experience limitations. A major life event took place when mom was forced to accept that she was no longer able to drive. Because of this she could not perform basic activities such as running errands or taking drives through the countryside. She missed her freedom to jump in the car and drive away to visit friends she left behind when she moved closer to her kids. Her sense of autonomy was significantly diminished. My mother was fiercely independent throughout her life. She completed two master's degrees while working full time and raising teenagers. She attended political and cultural events all over the California Bay Area and relied on old cars and trusty mechanics to help get her where she wanted to go.

There was a noticeable change in my mother's demeanor when she told us she was no longer able to drive. This shift reflected the grief she felt in saying goodbye to an important part of her life. It was gone forever. I also became aware of my mother's vulnerability. For the first time in my life, I began to think about the possibility of losing her.

Although the winter season of my mother's life brought challenges and emotions my siblings and I weren't prepared for, we also experienced gifts we could not have anticipated. Mom was home more, spending time reading and praying. The family often gathered to join in the seasonal abundance of warm soups and homemade breads. She seemed to become more introspective and began to think about writing her autobiography as she reflected on her achievements and challenges. I spent more time with her, engaging in lively conversations concerning politics and current events. I developed a deeper appreciation for her beautiful mind. During this time I was in my mid-40s. I felt challenges associated with the onset of menopause, while also experiencing a sense of accomplishment in my work and creative endeavors. The ability to join our lives together became a significant challenge as well as an opportunity to grow together. I recall a gentle transition into the springtime of my mother's life, a time of new beginnings and possibilities.

The season of spring was a time of self-reflection and moving inward to find new meanings in life. Mom started her autobiography and also worked on a poetry book, which she eventually self-published. Often when I arrived at her house, I found her sitting on her garden swing. I saw her connecting more to nature. She smiled at the hummingbirds gathering at the feeder, and she marveled in the beauty of the flowers blooming around her. Her life seemed less complicated yet much richer in many ways. I look back at the spring season of my mother's life with happiness and gratitude for all the gifts we shared during that time.

The summer season brought changes in my mom's perception of herself. She no longer identified as a professional woman in retirement. Rather, she tapped into the wisdom and experience that came with being a mother and grandmother. She gave us counsel that was meant to last a lifetime, not only for the immediate situation her children or grandchildren were experiencing. It was a subtle change, and not that noticeable until after her death when her words would come back, bringing comfort and hope.

Fall was the final and hardest season of mom's life. Although she maintained mental alertness until her death, she slowed down and often seemed to be in deep thought and was not as responsive as usual. Her physical movement was minimal and the people around her became her arms and legs. She was often frustrated and irritated. She had difficulty expressing her emotions. My mother had always been stoic and one day she told me, "I wish I could cry." This broke my heart.

I was determined to honor my mother's wish to stay at home until her death. I know that this is not always possible to do with an elderly parent, but I wanted to try. My siblings did not agree with my decision, and this led to fractures in my family that took time to mend. Five years later, we are still working on healing. I spent evenings with mom after long days of working and cared for her until her caregiver arrived. I received calls from providers during my workday and sometimes in the middle of the night. They needed to express their concerns and frustrations. It was not unusual for a caregiver to quit. I recall feeling overwhelmed, frustrated, and sad during the last two years of mom's life. I experienced incredible guilt for feeling this way. I also remember seeking joy and laughter whenever possible and this carried me through. In October 2019, my mother passed away peacefully at her home, in her bed. She died in the season she loved the most.

The moment my mother died, I felt her absence. I experienced an immediate loss of her energy, and it took my breath away. Our relationship was complicated, and we had differences of opinions and choices, but she was my anchor in this world, and I could go to her when I needed counsel or comfort. Since her death I have been fortunate to have other women in my life who bring friendship, love, and a deep sense of connection. I am so grateful for these relationships. Every time I go outside to walk, memories flood my mind and my mother is present. I see her in everything around me. I know that I am forever changed by her love, and all that she taught me about this life.

There is an art process I do which honors the life and death of my mother. It is a reminder that life as we know it comes to an end, but our mothers' lives can be remembered and celebrated. Then we can allow the process of letting-go to happen.

EXPLORATION: ART PROCESS

Cut a circle out of a piece of paper (or find a cardboard circle). Take the paper outside – to a place where you feel the presence of nature. Place the paper circle on the ground. Gather materials (e.g. leaves, sticks, rocks, etc.) and place them next to the circle. Using the gathered materials, create a design on the circle that represents your mother. Reflect on your creation and allow thoughts and feelings to come into your mind and heart. When you are finished, lift the circle and allow the materials to return to the earth.

REFERENCES

Behrman, S., & Crockett, C. (2024). Severe mental illness and the perimenopause. *BJPsych Bulletin*, 48(6), 364–370. https://doi.org/10.1192/bjb.2023.89

CBT-I International Directory. (2025). Perelman School of Medicine, University of Pennsylvania. https://cbti.directory/

Darpinian, S. (2022a, January 14). *Yoga therapy, asking for help, and avoiding the "all natural" mandate*. Therapy Rocks! https://audioboom.com/posts/8013305-yoga-therapy-asking-for-help-and-avoiding-the-all-natural-mandate

Darpinian, S. (2022b, October 1). *The New Science of Hope*. Therapy Rocks! https://audioboom.com/posts/8167409-the-new-science-of-hope

Darpinian, S. (2023, September 29). *The menopause brain and beyond*. Therapy Rocks! https://audioboom.com/posts/8376467-the-menopause-brain-and-beyond

Darpinian, S. (2024, September 30). *After Your Person Dies*. Therapy Rocks! https://audioboom.com/posts/8579784-after-your-person-dies

Edinger, J. D., & Carney, C. E. (2015). *Overcoming insomnia: A cognitive-behavioral therapy approach therapist guide* (2nd ed.). Oxford University Press.

Gunter, D. J. (2024, March 11). Depression, low mood and menopause [Substack newsletter]. *The Vajenda*. https://vajenda.substack.com/p/depression-low-mood-and-menopause

Harris, R. (2010). *A Quick Look at Your Values*. https://www.actmindfully.com.au/upimages/2016_Complete_Worksheets_for_Russ_Harris_ACT_Books.pdf

Hunter, M., & Smith, M. (2014). *Managing hot flushes and night sweats: A cognitive behavioural self-help guide to the menopause*. Routledge.

Krystal, A. D., Prather, A. A., & Ashbrook, L. H. (2019). The assessment and management of insomnia: An update. *World Psychiatry*, 18(3), 337–352. https://doi.org/10.1002/wps.20674

Lei, L., Leggett, A. N., & Maust, D. T. (2023). A national profile of sandwich generation caregivers providing care to both older adults and children. *Journal of the American Geriatrics Society*, 71(3), 799–809. https://doi.org/10.1111/jgs.18138

Makeba, W. (2024, September 10–14). *Mood, sleep, and cognitive function 101*. The Menopause Society Annual Meeting [Video recording]. https://watch.ondemand.org/player/30984/86482/sessions-630

Maki, P. M., & Jaff, N. G. (2022). Brain fog in menopause: A health-care professional's guide for decision-making and counseling on cognition. *Climacteric*, 25(6), 570–578. https://doi.org/10.1080/13697137.2022.2122792

Maki, P., & Jaff, N. (2024). *Menopause and brain fog: How to counsel and treat midlife women*. The Menopause Society: Practice Pearl. https://menopause.org/wp-content/uploads/professional/practice-pearl-brain-fog_a651c6e2-7190-4faf-ae7f-0d93bce0284f.pdf

Mosconi, L. (with Shriver, M.) (2024). *The menopause brain: New science empowers women to navigate the pivotal transition with knowledge and confidence* (1st ed.). Penguin Publishing Group.

Neufeld, S. (2018). *Awake at 3 a. M: Yoga therapy for anxiety and depression in pregnancy and early motherhood*. Parallax Press.

Santoro, N. (2024, September 10–14). *Vasomotor symptoms 101*. The Menopause Society Annual Meeting [Video recording]. https://watch.ondemand.org/player/30984/86475/sessions-630

Schmidt, P. J., Haq, N., & Rubinow, D.R. (2004). A longitudinal evaluation of the relationship between reproductive status and mood in perimenopausal women. *American Journal of Psychiatry*, 161(12), 2238–2244. https://doi.org/10.1176/appi.ajp.161.12.2238

Zhang, B., & Wing, Y.-K. (2006). Sex differences in insomnia: A meta-analysis. *Sleep*, 29(1), 85–93. https://doi.org/10.1093/sleep/29.1.85

Four

Providing Protective Factors for Disordered Eating in Midlife

Disordered eating that barely skirts the line between typical and problematic is highly common, more so than diagnosed eating disorders. Some signs of disordered eating are skipping meals, eating large amounts of food at one time, avoiding certain food groups, frequently dieting and weight cycling, feeling anxiety around food choices, and excessive exercising. These behaviors are so culturally sanctioned that they can sneak under the radar.

Menopause-fueled body changes can ignite disordered eating or an eating disorder, as well as ramp up long-standing behaviors that predate the menopause transition for some women. The body dissatisfaction from midlife changes can lead to wanting to "do something" to reverse the changes and alter appearance. A study found that 73 percent of midlife women experience dissatisfaction with their weight, which is a significant risk factor for the development of an eating disorder (Samuels et al., 2019).

The term disordered eating is often used to identify and describe some of the different eating behaviors that do not necessarily meet the diagnostic criteria for an eating disorder. It refers to a spectrum of problematic eating behaviors and distorted attitudes towards food, weight, shape, and appearance. The frequency, severity, and duration of symptoms determine where disordered eating ends and a clinical eating disorder begins. Both seriously impair quality of life and take up a lot of head space, making it difficult to be present.

At any given time, about two-thirds of menopausal women are dieting in midlife. Dieting is another leading risk factor for the development of a clinical eating disorder, and though not every woman who diets will develop an eating disorder, the development of a clinical

DOI: 10.4324/9781003632245-6

eating disorder typically starts with a diet. Unfortunately, it's not uncommon for doctors to prescribe intentional weight loss to women in midlife. This not only promotes anti-fat bias, it puts women at high risk for developing an eating disorder. Deb Burgard, a psychologist and activist specializing in weight stigma says, "We prescribe in fat people what we diagnose as disordered in thin people."

FOUR KEYS TO HEALTH AND VITALITY IN MIDLIFE AND BEYOND

by Jennifer L. Gaudiani, MD, CEDS-C, FAED

Margarita is a 52-year-old pharmacist whose last menstrual period was 14 months ago. Prior to this, she'd had three years of much heavier but less frequent periods. Starting around age 45, she felt like her body was going through a second adolescence, given all the changes she experienced at once. She suddenly started experiencing insomnia, where she'd wake up to pee at 3 a.m. and wouldn't get back to sleep because her thoughts were racing. Alcohol started to affect her mood and ability to get to sleep, so she had to cut back on what had been moderate drinking. Her mood on the whole worsened, and after resuming therapy productively, she did start on an antidepressant, which helped her feel more like herself. Hot flashes, while not as severe as some of her friends', have been frequent in the past two years.

Margarita has gone through cycles of dieting from college onward, and her weight has risen and dropped about 20 pounds many times over the years. As of age 45, she felt that her weight rose and stayed put, regardless of how she ate. Around her 50th birthday, she noticed her waist thickening in ways that weight had never distributed before and felt like her body was unfamiliar to her. She does cardio exercise when she can, but she's balancing work, two teenagers, and a recent divorce, so she often simply has no time. She hasn't wanted to do strength training because she worries about her body getting bigger. Margarita has found herself restricting calories more than she ever did and going down rabbit holes on the internet about weight loss. She certainly doesn't have the money to pay cash for one of the weight loss injectables everyone is talking about.

Half Mexican and half Caucasian, Margarita worries about her mom, who now has severe osteoporosis and has dealt with spine problems and a hip fracture. Margarita still isn't sure if she wants to go on menopause hormone therapy (MHT) despite no family history of breast cancer, because she has heard mixed reviews.

While people often focus on the development of eating disorders during adolescence, menopause is another important and common time when eating disorders may develop or recur (Davies, 2024; Vincent et al., 2024). Studies show that women at this time of life have a two to eight percent prevalence of developing a full DSM-5 eating disorder (Mangweth-Matzek et al., 2023). Complex psycho-social-medical transitions during this time can make midlife feel like a second adolescence. Women experience body composition changes, hormone fluctuations, vasomotor symptoms (hot flashes), mood changes, alterations in sex drive and function, having to attend both to one's older parents and children – especially as women start families at a later age – and aging in a society still hyper-focused on youth and thinness can all make a desire for control of food and body very compelling. This has been heightened by the "availability" (for those who can afford more than $1000/month) of injectable weight-loss medications.

The truth is that every woman will go through menopause uniquely, just like no two people's experience of adolescence is the same. For some it will be easy, and for others it will be chaotic and extremely difficult. Central and general weight gain during these years brings the physiologic benefit that fat cells become the sole producers of estrogen after the ovaries stop making it. This is important for bone density and sexual function. But because of the power of thin privilege and the megaphone of social media, women can be led into thinking that if they just try hard enough, they, too, can look like a 30-year-old at age 55. Some few may be able to do this (with a lot of cosmetic surgery or a lot of favorable genetics), but it simply isn't reasonable to expect of ourselves. That said, there are a number of wonderfully beneficial ways we can support our health during these years.

First of all, women during perimenopause and menopause may benefit from MHT. Research has shown that besides improving quality of life by treating bothersome symptoms, MHT can reduce your risk for CVD and metabolic disease, including insulin resistance. MHT can also reduce your risk of bone fractures and osteoporosis.

Next up: Strength training – exercise using body weight against gravity, using resistance bands, or using weights to improve muscle strength – has been shown to result in vital improvements in cardiovascular, bone, and metabolic health (Momma et al., 2022). I refer to muscle mass as a "glucose sponge" because it helps so much with insulin sensitivity. If we can think about physical activity not as a means to weight loss (because it isn't) but as a means to vitality, independence, and self-care, then it's much easier to do consistently. In the Oslo Ischemia Study, for instance, participants who improved their physical activity dropped their mortality risk by a third and their stroke risk by 60 percent, with no changes in body mass index (Prestgaard et al., 2019). Both cardio and strength training are wonderful for the body. However, how we look as a result of exercise is mostly dependent on our genetics.

Third, bone density will stay strongest with exercise, MHT (if needed for low bone mass, or high risk for osteoporosis), and great nutrition. Undernourishment decreases bone density formation, and with increased menopausal bone resorption, dieting and eating disorder behaviors can swiftly cause fragile bones.

Finally, being as kind and compassionate and accepting of our bodies as possible is the best way to approach these years. I know society makes that incredibly challenging, but it's true. How many of us have asked, looking at gorgeous (if awkward) teenage photos of ourselves, "How could I have spent so much time being miserable about my body at that age? I was adorable!" I can assure you: Our future 80-year-old selves would say the same thing to us now. Long years of maintaining too-low a body weight, or cycles of dieting, all set us up to gain more weight in menopause. Nutritionally the best and most scientifically-rigorous choice is to care for your body as if you plan to rely on it for another 40–50 years (because you will!), drop the dieting, and eat consistently and satisfyingly.

DISORDERED EATING AND EATING DISORDERS

Eating disorders have the second highest mortality rate of any psychiatric illness behind opiate addiction (Arcelus et al., 2011). When I started treating disordered eating and eating disorders 25 years ago, people were more straightforward about the diets they were on for intentional weight loss. In a discovery call about my services they would say things like, "I went on Jenny Craig to try to lose weight and I think it's morphed into an eating disorder."

Today, the most common thing I hear on these calls is, "I just want to lose weight in a healthy way." On one hand, people are more informed about eating disorders, but as wellness culture has seeped into diet culture, the desire to lose weight in the name of "health" sneaks under the radar. We are so inundated with diet culture messaging, it makes sense that people associate "thin" with "healthy." Contrary to popular belief, undereating, restricting certain food groups, developing anxiety around food, and exercising in ways that are not nutritionally supported do not improve health – they are signs of disordered eating. If you recognize these behaviors in yourself, it might be time to seek support.

As you saw in the preface, diets have a 95–98 percent failure rate. Not only do people gain their weight back, they typically gain to a higher weight than before the diet. People are left feeling like failures, and like they failed at their diet, but the reality is that the diet is failing them. This is how the diet industry is going strong at $72 billion. Says Shilo George, "Intentional weight loss is like gambling; the house always wins."

A study that investigated the lifetime/12-month prevalence of eating disorders (EDs) amongst women in mid-life (i.e., fourth and fifth decade of life) found that 15.3 percent of women have met criteria for a lifetime ED. The 12-month prevalence of EDs was 3.6 percent. The study found that only 27 percent of midlife women who met criteria for a clinical eating disorder received treatment or sought help (Micali et al., 2017). Why is this? The reasons are multifactorial, but stereotypes such as that eating disorders exist in straight, white, affluent girls (an acronym called SWAG), lead to overlooking underrecognized populations including, but not limited to, women in midlife and beyond (*Eating Disorder Myths*, 2025). I read somewhere that treating an eating disorder is like fighting a forest fire, you cannot leave an ember smoldering. Midlife is full of stressful embers. Cynthia M. Bulik, PhD, founding director of the University of North Carolina Center of Excellence for Eating Disorders says, "When I was 18 years old, I broke my back. And though my back is fully healed, I have a vulnerability. I will never do things like bungee jumping. I want to honor my health legacy." She went on to say, "Full recovery from an eating disorder is possible, but it's not without its vulnerabilities, it's part of your health legacy. We have to honor our health legacies."

Bulik and her team at the UNC Center of Excellence for Eating Disorders conducted the largest-ever research study of genetic and environmental causes of eating disorders. Three years ago Bulik's team identified eight regions on the genome associated with anorexia nervosa (AN). Their genetic analyses also showed that both psychiatric and metabolic factors influenced risk for developing AN. They suggested that AN be considered a metabo-psychiatric disorder. AN is an illness she says we have "psychologized" for decades. Individuals with this particular eating disorder have a "paradoxical response to a negative energy balance." In lay terms, this means that these individuals can sustain under-eating, whether it's intentional or not. It's not typically as uncomfortable for them to undereat, which is unusual given that feeding ourselves is essential for our survival.

Individuals experiencing a robust recovery from AN need to be "religious" about not ever getting into a negative energy balance through undereating or dieting. This is an example of honoring their health legacy. This is easier said than done. I've had clients with a history of AN who are in a robust recovery from their eating disorder, and then go on a trip to Europe. On the trip they might be expending more energy than usual from trekking around, with less access to food because of traveling, and unintentionally end up in a negative energy balance. Bulik's team says this puts them at risk biologically (and psychologically) of falling into that negative energy balance spiral. The body pulls itself back down in weight, wanting to revert to a negative settling point.

Dieting and intentional weight loss are about intentionally engaging in a negative energy balance, which is risky business for anyone, especially those with a history of an eating disorder. In addition, we have to contend with weight cycling, which is the process of going on a diet, losing weight, and then regaining the weight (and sometimes more). This leads to changes in metabolism, binge eating, preoccupation with food and inflammation, and also often leads to a higher weight than an individual would be at naturally without a history of gaining and losing.

THE DEPRIVE/DEVOUR CYCLE

As a therapist working with disordered eating and eating disorders, I need to know a fair amount about the dietitian's role, just as they need to know about the mental health aspects of treatment. So when a client comes to me initially stating, "I find myself doing a lot of stress eating during the day and especially at night," it's clear they will need to be more grounded in their food and routines before they are ready to eat in an attuned way. When clients initially seek help for their eating difficulties, and report feeling out of control with their food, I try to get a feel for whether or not they are in a deprive/devour cycle.

A deprive/devour cycle might look like eating too little during the day, which sets them up to overeat at night. They blame themselves for overeating and don't recognize it's often because they aren't eating enough during the day. They say, "I am definitely eating enough, that's not the problem, it's that I'm eating too much." People believe they are eating enough, but they are so immersed in diet culture that it's rare that their self reporting is accurate. I will ask them to describe what a typical day of eating is like, or more specifically, ask them to provide the specifics of what they ate the day before. I can often tell when there are gaps in their intake, or missed meals, which lead to overeating. In other words, their overeating at night won't stop until they start eating more throughout the day.

If the above is the case, I refer to a Registered Dietitian (RD) who is also a Certified Eating Disorder Specialist (CEDS), with a weight-inclusive, non-diet approach. This kind of referral, if it is accessible to a client, can accelerate healing and recovery, and allows me as the therapist to stay within my scope of practice.

"I always assess their ABC's: is their diet Adequate (A), Balanced (B), and Consistent (C)," says Registered Dietitian Wendy Sterling, MS, RD, CSSD, CEDS-C and co-author of *How to Nourish Yourself Through an Eating Disorder: Recovery for Adults with the Plate-by-Plate Approach*. She explains that she will assess whether her clients are eating adequately enough to meet their energy needs (including to fuel the frequency, duration, and intensity of their exercise). This usually includes three full meals and at least two snacks.

"Most forget about snacks…but snacks are important for boosting energy, metabolism, and helping to maintain blood sugar levels throughout the day," Sterling says. She will also review the nutritional balance of a client's diet by looking at whether they are including all food groups. Carbohydrates, proteins, fruits, vegetables, fats, and calcium rich foods, all play an important role in our health. And finally, are they doing all of these things consistently throughout the day, week, and weekend?

Stabilizing one's food patterns requires putting full meals together, regularly and consistently. This can be hard for many of our patients who are used to dieting and eating as little as possible at meals. Clients will often say, "I'm hesitant to eat this much, it's bringing up all of this stuff for me." They fear they are going to gain weight, when they want to lose it. This is certainly understandable, given we live in a society where weight stigma (the devaluation of an individual based on body weight or body shape) is rampant. As much as people find it difficult to tolerate the uncertainty about where their body is going to land when eating adequately, they also want out of the deprive/devour cycle they've been in for years. They want to be in their lives, and as they approach midlife, they become much more uncomfortable with the headspace this cycle takes up.

HELEN'S STORY

Helen had come to therapy as she entered late postmenopause because she was tired of yo-yo dieting. She came to me saying she couldn't recall a time in her life ever feeling comfortable in her body. In her early twenties she likely had undiagnosed binge-eating disorder, or BED. BED is characterized by recurrent episodes of binge eating and eating larger amounts of food in a discrete period of time than most people would in the same situation. She used food as a way to cope with her abusive relationship; food was her inventive adaptation for survival. Once she entered her thirties, Helen joined Overeaters Anonymous (OA), which encouraged her to restrict certain food groups, using the addiction model. She believed she couldn't trust herself around food, and OA's paradigm kept this story alive.

Helen, tired of the deprive/devour cycle, sought my services to lay down dieting once and for all. I explained, as do many of us using a weight-inclusive, non-diet approach, that when we start to use the trust model – getting back to what our bodies already know how to do – we might gain weight, lose weight or stay the same. This is not exactly a "sexy sell" in a culture that idolizes youth and thinness! Helen consented to this work. I made a referral to a non-diet dietitian, with whom Helen worked on debunking the diet myths she had believed for so long, and started to build trust around the foods she was made to believe she couldn't have. This resulted in her natural weight.

One marker of our natural weight, also known as our "set-point weight," is the weight we return to in between diets (Bacon & Aphramor, 2014). But what if you don't like your body's natural weight? Of course we all have body autonomy, and adults can certainly engage in intentional weight loss, should they choose. A non-diet/weight inclusive approach is too much of a paradigm shift for some. One of the problems, however, is that many people are "choosing" intentional weight loss without proper informed consent; they don't have a comprehensive understanding of the risks and benefits associated with intentional weight loss. Val Schonberg, RD, CSSD, MSCP states, "In the late perimenopause timeframe we see an increased decline in bone density, then it tapers off to about .5 percent per year. It would be in our best interest to not do anything to contribute to this loss. Every time we lose weight we lose bone mass and lean tissue (which is our muscle). When people gain the weight back it gets gained back as fat. We can't get the bone back, so this weight cycling leads to bone loss" (Darpinian, 2023).

"When you restrict your food and/or make certain foods off limits, it leads to overeating or bingeing on the foods you aren't allowing yourself to have. This feels compulsive, but compulsion is not the same as bona fide addiction," says Marci Evans MS, CEDS-C, LDN.

Once food gets recalibrated, and you add back in foods you have been avoiding, you can start to eat in response to what your body is calling for, and the bingeing will start to level out.

Evans continues:

> There is evidence that individuals have an amplified neurobiological response to highly processed foods (as compared to minimally processed foods), but that response is complicated to understand, because a wide variety of factors such as dietary restriction, internalized weight bias, poor body image, and a history of dieting can all contribute to what we see happening in the brains, bodies, and behaviors of people. Extreme dietary approaches to manage feelings of food addiction are not sustainable and actually worsen feelings of food addiction for most people.

FIVE STAGES OF CHANGE: DISORDERED EATING AND EATING DISORDERS

Psychologist James O. Prochaska developed The 5 Stages of Change model in the 1980s to promote awareness of how people change. I did a professional onsite visit to an eating disorder residential program, where I attended a workshop by Hunter Taylor, presenting his adapted version of the 5 Stages using more recovery language. Hunter, a Licensed Clinical Psychotherapist, did his workshop on the stages through drama therapy, having clinicians from the audience act out the stages.

The body language of Stage One, "Denial," was arms folded, demonstrating resistance. In this stage people don't see their current behavior as a problem. In the case of disordered eating, it's so pervasive in our culture it's hard for people to see it as a problem. Often, they are often praised for their weight loss efforts and diets.

A client of mine said, "When I was in Stage One, 'Denial,' it was because I thought I had my disordered eating for so long that I couldn't change, and I wasn't ready to give up restricting my food."

When the actors were acting out Stage Two, "Contemplation," they had their hand on their chin, and a facial expression of someone who looked as though they were in a state of deciding. Contemplation is not being sure. An individual might start to see evidence of a problem with dieting/disordered eating at this stage, but is not certain whether it is serious enough to do something different. Some people are in this stage for a long time. They are considering change, but are on the fence with it, or on the defensive with it.

You might hear a person in this stage say, "Well, I have been dieting my whole life, and nothing has ever worked to sustain my weight loss. It does take up a lot of head space, but I don't think I could ever be okay with my natural weight."

In Stage Three, the clinicians in the drama therapy skit threw their hands up in the air to demonstrate the third stage, "Surrender." In this stage people say, "Tell me what I need to do, I'm tired of suffering." There are more pros than cons at this point. This is a stage of skills acquisition to learn more about why diets don't work, as well as to learn about alternatives to dieting. Hunter notes, "Fear is often what stands between Surrender and the next stage, Action. The fear is to lose one's identity of being in the problem, and the risk of stepping into change. Some are at an impasse with Surrender. They acknowledge they have a problem but are resistant to change, as they don't know who they are without the problem." In relation to disordered eating/eating disorders, the fear of recovery is often related to the fear of gaining weight and a changing body.

A client said, "When I was in Surrender, I wanted to be done with the deprive/devour cycle I was in. I understood the nutrition science I was learning in my work with a dietitian, and how my undereating was leading to binges. But I feared weight gain, and the loss of the external validation I received from people about how young and fit I looked in my late 50s, when the reality was that I was in an active eating disorder that was ruining my life."

Action, Stage Four is about applying what you know. The actors were "running in place" for this one, an active stage of change. This might look like taking the psycho education about diets and actively applying a more calibrated approach such as the ABCs we talked about earlier in the chapter, as well as getting more support through therapy and a non-diet dietitian.

The same client has now increased her support with her dietitian, and is engaging in her new way of eating more often than her old one. She rarely binges, has habituated to her body changes, and is overall much more present and happy in her life.

Stage Five, Maintenance, is the last stage. There's habit formation here. Individuals are no longer using food restriction or binging as a way to cope. They are eating in a more embodied way, occasionally getting activated and moving backwards to another stage.

EXPLORATION: THE FIVE STAGES OF CHANGE

Where are you in the stages below? Describe the stage you're in with as much detail as possible.

Stage One: Denial

No need to seek a solution because people feel there isn't a problem. Limited awareness, or lack insight into the consequences of negative behavior. More cons than pros related to changing a behavior. Not common to seek treatment at this stage.

Stage Two: Contemplation

The problem sits center stage, in a state of deciding. Weighing out the pros/cons.

Stage Three: Surrender

More pros for changing than cons, information-gathering stage. To surrender would mean giving up an identity. Fear of stepping into the unknown.

Stage Four: Action

Moving into change, getting support. It's an active state, where the person starts to apply what they know.

Stage Five: Maintenance

Habit formation has occurred. The individual has replaced the old behaviors with new behaviors most of the time. If they go backwards to another stage there's typically a quick return to their baseline behaviors.

REFERENCES

Arcelus, J., et al. (2011). "Mortality rates in patients with anorexia nervosa and other eating disorders. A meta-analysis of 36 studies." *Archives of General Psychiatry* 68(7), 724–731. https://doi.org/10.1001/archgenpsychiatry.2011.74

Bacon, L., & Aphramor, L. (2014). *Body respect: What conventional health books get wrong, leave out, and just plain fail to understand about weight*. BenBella Books, Inc.

Darpinian, S. (2023, November 28). Menopause, nutrition, and diet culture: Getting the facts straight on midlife health. Episode 40. *Therapy Rocks!* https://audioboom.com/posts/8408208-menopause-nutrition-and-diet-culture-getting-the-facts-straight-on-midlife-health

Davies, H. O. (2024). Eating disorders of the perimenopause. *Post Reproductive Health*, 30(4), 233–238. https://doi.org/10.1177/20533691241293905

Eating Disorder Myths: What You Need to Know. (2025). Project HEAL. Retrieved May 24, 2025, from https://www.theprojectheal.org/common-misconceptions-about-eating-disorders-people-who-have-them-stereotype-vs-reality

Mangweth-Matzek, B., Kummer, K. K., & Hoek, H. W. (2023). Update on the epidemiology and treatment of eating disorders among older people. *Current Opinion in Psychiatry*, 36(6), 405–411. https://doi.org/10.1097/YCO.0000000000000893

Micali, N., Martini, M. G., Thomas, J. J., Eddy, K. T., Kothari, R., Russell, E., Bulik, C. M., & Treasure, J. (2017). Lifetime and 12-month prevalence of eating disorders amongst women in mid-life: A population-based study of diagnoses and risk factors. *BMC Medicine*, 15(1), 12. https://doi.org/10.1186/s12916-016-0766-4

Momma, H., Kawakami, R., Honda, T., & Sawada, S. S. (2022). Muscle-strengthening activities are associated with lower risk and mortality in major non-communicable diseases: A systematic review and meta-analysis of cohort studies. *British Journal of Sports Medicine*, 56(13), 755–763. https://doi.org/10.1136/bjsports-2021-105061

Prestgaard, E., Mariampillai, J., Engeseth, K., Erikssen, J., Bodegård, J., Liestøl, K., Gjesdal, K., Kjeldsen, S., Grundvold, I., & Berge, E. (2019). Change in cardiorespiratory fitness and risk of stroke and death: Long-term follow-up of healthy middle-aged men. *Stroke*, 50(1), 155–161. https://doi.org/10.1161/STROKEAHA.118.021798

Samuels, K. L., Maine, M. M., & Tantillo, M. (2019). Disordered eating, eating disorders, and body image in midlife and older women. *Current Psychiatry Reports*, 21(8), 70. https://doi.org/10.1007/s11920-019-1057-5

Vincent, C., Bodnaruc, A. M., Prud'homme, D., Guenette, J., & Giroux, I. (2024). Disordered eating behaviours during the menopausal transition: A systematic review. *Applied Physiology, Nutrition, and Metabolism*, 49(10), 1286–1308. https://doi.org/10.1139/apnm-2023-0623

PART 3
Diet-Free Living

Eating in Response to the Body's Wisdom

Five

The menopause transition can lead to changes in weight and redistribution, leaving women looking for solutions. The real solution lies in our health behaviors, and weight is not a behavior (given that trying to modify it rarely works). Handling stress, being in the habit of moving, developing and maintaining healthy relationships, getting good sleep, and eating to appetite are examples of health behaviors. These are the same if you are living in a larger body, a smaller one, or somewhere in the middle.

In Chapter 4, we broke down why diets don't work, and how they can make people feel hopeless. Often my clients say, "If I can't diet, then what am I going to do?"

In this chapter we are going to focus on an alternative to dieting. For some, it will simply validate what you're already doing, and maybe add some new tools to your toolbox as you enter menopause and the body starts speaking a different language. For others, these ideas might seem radical after years of dieting according to others' rules. (This is called an external locus of control – when you rely on someone else, such as an influencer or fad diet, to tell you when and/or what to eat. This is a slippery slope, because it creates a relationship to food that's reliant on everything happening in a controlled setting and functioning "perfectly.") In this scenario a client might say, "I wish my co-workers wouldn't bring cupcakes to work. If they're there I'll eat them, if they're not, I won't."

Conversely, an internal locus of control comes from a place of self trust around food. It's knowing you can have cupcakes any time you want them; they're not off limits. You can take this internal locus of control anywhere with you, so for example when you arrive at work

DOI: 10.4324/9781003632245-8

and see cupcakes, your decision to eat one (or not) comes from a place of embodiment. You might decide from the inside and ask yourself, "Am I hungry?" "Do I like this kind of cupcake?" You could even think, "I just ate breakfast, but a cupcake sounds fun and I'd like to celebrate Tasha's birthday." Bottom line, you're not giving power to a cupcake that it doesn't have. Your decision comes from a place of personal potency.

Developing our internal locus is one of many ways we can harness and nurture our own intuitive reflexes and best thinking. We often hear mixed messages in the menopause space regarding our ability to make decisions for ourselves. On one hand there is a lot written about the wisdom that comes from accumulated life experience in midlife and beyond, but on the other hand I see just as much written about not being able to trust our own appetites, leaving us thinking, "I can finally trust myself now that I have all this wisdom, but I still can't trust my own body." You are to be trusted, and below are some skills and tools to cultivate that self trust.

SELF INQUIRY

Before you read on, it's important to understand the evolution of your relationship with food. What messages did you receive about food in your home? What was happening in the culture at large? Are there ways you'd like to be feeling, thinking and behaving differently as it relates to your relationship to food? If you were coming of age in the 1980s like I was, you probably remember the fat-free diet era. This particular fad diet illuminated the importance of satisfaction in our relationship to food. We tried to eat "fat free," and I distinctly remember my mom eating entire packages of rice cakes, chasing the satisfaction she was never going to get, leaving her endlessly unsatisfied.

Second, if the evolution of things for you, as it relates to food, involves a history of chronic dieting, introducing satisfaction and pleasure might be activating at first. It's not uncommon for me to hear people say things like, "I can't bring yummy things into the house, that's all I'd eat." You might be right initially. But if one of the ways you'd like to feel differently about your relationship to food is to use less headspace around it, you'll need to include all foods in your diet, not just those deemed healthy. Once all fare is fair, you'll be able to discern what your body is calling for, versus what you're not allowing yourself to have.

PREREQUISITES FOR EATING IN RESPONSE TO THE BODY'S WISDOM

There are a few things to consider before someone is ready to eat in a more attuned way. First, are they getting seven to nine hours of sleep each night, the recommended amount for an adult? This matters because sleep deficiency causes increased production of ghrelin, which generates sensations of hunger and decreased production of leptin, which promotes satiety. Secondly, if an individual has an active eating disorder, eating intuitively would be premature until they are weight restored and in a robust recovery. A history of a restrictive eating disorder, such as Anorexia Nervosa, as well as neurodivergence, may predispose an individual to a lack of interoceptive awareness (the ability to be aware of internal sensations such as hunger and fullness). Eating to appetite may need to look more mechanical for some populations. An example of mechanical eating is eating by the clock on the wall instead of in response to internal cues. This sounds simple but it's not easy to eat without hunger. Nevertheless, this is an important skill to strengthen, especially for those in a robust recovery from an eating disorder or disordered eating. Finally, there are certain medications that tend to disembody people from their hunger and fullness cues; their intuitive eating might also look more like eating at certain times.

Factors That Make It Difficult to Hear What Your Body Is Saying

An active eating disorder
High stress
Bereavement
Mood disruption
A divorce or major life event
Sickness
Medications
Caffeine
Recreational drugs and alcohol

HUNGER METER

One of the most helpful tools for fine tuning hunger and fullness cues is the Hunger Meter (HM) (see Figure 5.1). It's a tool that helps create awareness and cultivate curiosity between you and your food. In the beginning, when you feel a pull toward food, simply press the pause button and ask yourself where you are on the HM before eating. It's a great way to get back to eating in a more embodied way, especially if your food choices historically have been made from the "chin up." That said, the HM isn't a perfect tool for everyone, especially if you have limited interoceptive awareness and are unable to access your hunger and satiety cues.

In my previous book, *Raising Body Positive Teens: A Parent's Guide to Diet-Free Living, Exercise, and Body Image*, my co-authors and I wrote extensively about using the HM.

> If you are ready to begin learning to assess your hunger and fullness, this tool is a great place to start. Keep in mind that to keep your body's metabolism on track, you should be diving into that initial meal within the first hour of getting up. It's important to keep your metabolism alert and operational by eating regularly throughout the day. Eating every three to four hours is a good way to teach yourself to feel hungry throughout the day, while preventing you from feeling ravenous later on. For example, let's say you wake up at 7 a.m. Perhaps breakfast is at 7.30. Depending

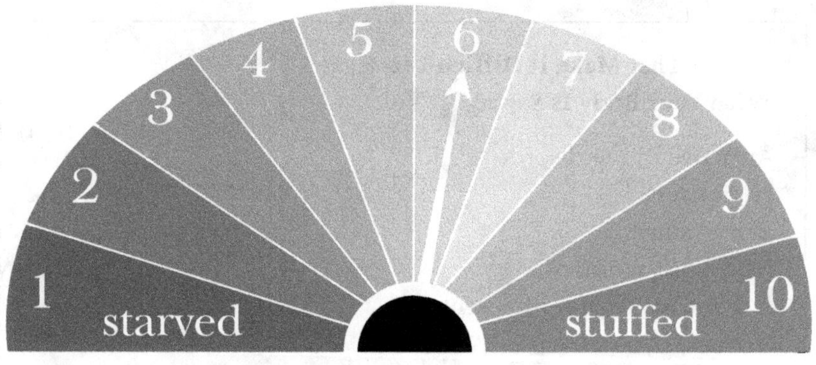

Figure 5.1 The Hunger Meter

> on what time you have lunch, you might need a snack mid-morning at 9.30, when your stomach starts rumbling. Aim for lunch by noon, snack at 3 p.m., dinner at 6, and an evening snack at 9.
>
> (Darpinian, 2022, p. 108)

The HM uses a scale of 1–10 with gradations of hunger to fullness. When you're getting started just tune in and see if you can *decide from the inside* where you are on the Hunger Meter before you eat.

Hunger Meter: From Starving to Stuffed

- 1 = Ravenous, dizzy, cranky, can't think clearly, low blood sugar
- 2 = Very hungry, rumbling stomach
- 3 = Manageable hunger, a happy place where you want to arrive at mealtime, calm and mindful about eating
- 4 = You could eat, but you're not that hungry; snacky
- 5 = You've probably just eaten and aren't hungry
- 6 = A stopping place with room for more; your stomach feels happy and at peace, but it's not overly stuffed
- 7 = Your taste buds lose interest much beyond this point
- 8 = You are on the path toward full and feel anchored by your food
- 9 = Thanksgiving Day stuffed
- 10 = Time to pull on the PJ pants

> Ultimately, the key is to match your fuel to your hunger level. For example, if you are a 4, you might need a small snack, such as fruit with a small handful of nuts. If you are a 1 on the HM – that is, basically starving – you probably need a full meal. Just an apple will not do. As your blood sugar comes back to normal, ask yourself, "Why was I so hungry? Did I miss something that day? Was my lunch not filling enough?
>
> (Darpinian, 2022, p. 111)

> Whether it's time for a meal or snack, it's recommended to arrive at a manageable hunger, or a 3 on the HM – the first sign of hunger. You feel calm and mindful about the decision to eat. You're not ravenous, but you may feel a little twinge in your stomach, a little emptiness telling you that your body wants food. It's been a few hours since you had your last meal, and you feel ready to find food so your brain and body can perform at an optimum level. Factors including what taste, texture, and

temperature of food you are in the mood for (these are called the 3 Ts) – sweet, smooth, creamy, crunchy, hot, or warm – can help you figure out what to eat. This is important because being "satisfied" with your food selection is tied to your stopping place.

(Darpinian, 2022, p. 111)

CAN'T I JUST FOCUS ON "HEALTHY EATING" AND BE FINE?

Satisfaction is nuanced as it relates to food. Feeling "satisfied" after a meal is both emotional and physical. It starts with where you are on the hunger meter when you begin eating. If you are at "3" on the HM (AKA "manageable hunger") making that decision will have a peaceful quality to it, allowing you to to tune in and decide from the inside what you want to eat. Starting at a "3" will also make it easier to stop at just enough (a "6" on the HM).

In the beginning, it's helpful to use the 3 T's when making a decision about what to eat, by taking an inventory on what "taste, texture, temperature" you want your food to be. If you are craving a burger, but tell yourself you need to have a protein bar instead "because it's healthy," you might be satisfied physically, but not emotionally. A person can feel the physical sensation of fullness without feeling the emotional and psychological pleasure of satisfaction. We need and crave both. When we think about the foods we tell ourselves we can't have, this is an example of the food noise diet culture creates. Incorporating satisfaction into your food choices quiets food noise, making it easier to stop at just enough. We are watching ourselves act, so when we make a food choice intuitively, and honor our cravings, we start to build self trust. We start to relax, knowing we can have a burger anytime we want. Right now is not your last chance. This will give you access to what your body is calling for versus what you aren't allowing yourself to have.

Restriction creates a physiological kind of food noise. Deprivation creates the drive for food; it's the way we are wired for survival. Of course, that noise will become louder the lower we get on the HM. The hungrier we get (1 or 2 on HM), the more the hunger hormone ghrelin increases, and leption (the hormone responsible for satiety) decreases. In other words, if the signal is loud the body's response will be loud.

BUILDING SELF TRUST AROUND FOOD

If you find yourself overly responding to certain foods, the first step is to make sure you are eating Adequately (A), Balanced (B), and Consistent (C) (ABCs) to reduce the internal vulnerability of getting too hungry. The second step is to have the "yummy foods" outside of the home, with a Cope Ahead plan in place. Cope Ahead is a DBT skill that's meant to be started before an anxiety producing event, increasing the likelihood you'll be able to use your skill in real time. You start first by identifying potential triggers so that they lose their potency, then you rehearse new emotional responses. People report feeling less blindsided by anxiety-producing events when using this skill.

COPE AHEAD

Practice ahead of time increases the chances of performing a desired skill or behavior (see Figure 5.2). Think of an event (large or small) that you're planning to attend. First, write down all of the potential "triggers" you think you might experience at the event (they lose some of their potency when you identify them). Then, list some new

Potential Triggers	New Emotional Responses
Getting too hungry before having a piece of pie, a 1 or 2 on the HM.	I will focus on eating adequate (A), balanced (B), and consistent (C) (ABCs) meals throughout the day today to ensure I have "manageable hunger" (a 3 on the HM) when it's time for pie.
As I'm eating the pie, I often tell myself that I'll need to restrict my food the rest of the day if I have a slice.	There's nothing wrong with pie, it can be a perfectly normal part of my relationship to food. If I restrict my food, I will end up overeating.
If I allow myself to eat pie, it's all I'm going to want to eat.	I might crave pie more often in the beginning because I have deemed it "off limits" in the past. Avoiding off limits foods maintains my fear around them. I am committed to heading toward these fear foods to give myself an opportunity to find that the fear is unfounded.
I always tell myself I'll only have one or two bites, then I end up eating the whole thing.	As I work on buliding self-trust around pie, I will commit to going out for a slice with a friend. I'll practice arriving at a 3, identifying the taste, temperature, and texture (3Ts) I'd like, and giving myself permission to eat it. I'll repeat the mantra, "There's more where that came from, I can have pie anytime I want."

Figure 5.2 Sample Cope Ahead Worksheet

and/or alternative emotional responses. It works best if you write out this skill a few days ahead.

Let's say pie is a food you'd like to build more trust around so you can ultimately bring a pie into the house without overly responding to it. Step one is identifying triggers and rehearsing new emotional responses.

Step two is imagining how well it could possibly go: You order the exact pie you want, you give yourself permission to eat the pie and savor it, stopping at a place that feels comfortable to you. Imagine leaving the restaurant with a sense of self mastery: "Yeah, I can do this!" Visualize being fully present with your friend and also being present while eating the piece of pie, so you don't miss the pleasure. At first it will be hard to know when pleasure ends and overeating begins – that's why we are setting up one piece of pie initially. Typically, "the mind wants to keep going even though the body is done." Mantras speak to your cells, "There's more where this came from, I can have pie anytime I want."

One more note on satisfaction. It's personal. You get to decide what satisfaction feels like to you. For example, you might not need your lunch to be as satisfying as your dinner. For lunch in the middle of a work day, you might eat more for utility and efficiency. You may want to eat in a way that leaves you feeling energized after your meal. Whereas at dinner, the satisfaction element might become more important to you, and you might want to feel a bit more anchored by your food after a meal, (AKA an "8" on the HM). The bottom line is that there's no way to get it wrong. If you are eating in a way that you can get wrong, you are likely on a diet (this excludes nutritionally sensitive diseases of course).

When feeling a pull toward food when you are full (an 8 to 10 on the HM), the focus is not so much on whether or not you end up eating the food, but more about creating space between you and the food to get a little more information. Did you not eat enough earlier in the day? Are you overly responding to a food that's previously been off limits to you? Are you feeding something else, like exhaustion or boredom? Creating the space between you and food is the skill to strengthen, in other words it's the "target behavior," which, if addressed, will create the most amount of change in your relationship to food.

MAKING FOOD EQUAL IN AVAILABILITY

Early in my career I distinctly remember having client sessions back to back for hours at a time, with ten minute breaks in between. My office was a craftsman style house converted into an office, complete with a full kitchen. One year, around Halloween, I noticed that when I had a chance to run into the kitchen during a break to grab food, I'd peer into the fridge and see a bag of Halloween candy as well as the "makings" for a sandwich. I'd typically be at a 1 or a 2 on the Hunger Meter, and grab what was easiest (the candy), versus what my body was actually calling for (the sandwich). I suddenly realized the importance of not only making foods equal in morality, but also equal in availability.

The point isn't that candy is bad or a sandwich is good, but that without proper planning you might gulp down whatever is quickest, instead of what your body actually needs. The goal is to have a fridge full of foods you know your body does really well with, but also to feel calm and grounded when you'd like candy (not frantic or impulsive, but a calm 3–4 on the Hunger Meter). Making food equal in availability requires preparation, and you are not always going to have time for the preliminary work required here. That's okay! It's all trial and error, there's no way to get it wrong. The goal is to cultivate curiosity on a day you didn't pack enough food, and notice how it sets you up to be ravenous when you get home. Log the info you need so that you can pack your food in a way that honors your future self (Darpinian, 2022, p. 117).

WHAT ABOUT SUGAR?

In my practice I'm often decoding the psychological aspects of food with the women in my caseload. It's not uncommon to have clients come into my practice thinking they have a problem with sugar. Of course I'm not suggesting "overconsumption of sugar" is a good thing, overconsumption of any one thing is not ideal. After I have a chance to tease things out over time, these are the most common themes I find:

- A pattern of getting too hungry. When we get too hungry our hunger hormone (ghrelin) rises, and the hormone that lets us know when we are sated (leptin) decreases. The body will then have strong cravings for the quickest source of energy: Sugar.

- The second most common pattern I see is people overly responding to the foods they aren't allowing themselves to have. Off limits foods create "food noise," the byproduct of diet culture. Once we work in therapy together to "legalize" all foods, that permission naturally leads to more moderate consumption.
- And theoretically, once all "fare is fair," the body/mind can crave what it needs versus what we aren't allowing it to have. In other words, forbidden fruit is the sweetest.

Interestingly, there are studies of women and chocolate cake. The women in the study who reported feeling guilty about eating chocolate cake reported lower levels of perceived behavioral control over eating cake and were less successful at maintaining their weight compared to those who associated chocolate cake with celebration (Kuijer & Boyce, 2014). Anecdotally, the women in my caseload report that not allowing themselves to have a prototypical forbidden food item, such as chocolate cake, leads to overly responding to the cake (eating more of it), as well as eating cake they don't even like. In other words, eating it "just because it's there."

You might be in need of repairing your relationship to sugar, but getting rid of sugar can lead to disordered eating, and further, it's not necessary.

- Finally, I find that some people use sweets, or other "treat" foods when they are in need of increasing their pleasant activities. It's a pattern I see with people who don't have a work/life balance, so eating sweets is the only "sweetness" they are giving themselves. This is an example of "decoding" their food choices. Of course, eating sweets is a perfectly normal part of a peaceful relationship to food, we just don't want it to be the *only* source of pleasure in our lives.

GENTLE NUTRITION IN MIDLIFE

by Jenn Salib Huber, RD, ND, CIEC

Midlife is often a time when women are told they need to overhaul everything, cut sugar, eliminate carbs, drink green sludge, and track every bite of food. But from an intuitive eating perspective, those external pressures are exactly the kind of noise that makes it hard to hear our internal cues. Gentle nutrition, instead, asks, "What do I want *and* what do I need?" It's okay (and expected) for the answer to shift from day to day. Sometimes that might mean prioritizing fiber to support digestion or lowering cholesterol. Other times, it might mean choosing something comforting because you're emotionally exhausted.

Once someone has built a foundation of attunement that includes sleeping enough, managing stress, nourishing regularly, and beginning to decode diet culture's food rules, they may feel ready to layer in gentle nutrition. This isn't about moralizing food or labeling meals as "good" or "bad," but rather about weaving in supportive choices that align with how they want to feel. In midlife, this can mean including foods that support bone health, heart health, and brain health, such as calcium-rich foods, fiber-filled plants or Omega-3 fats. It's a flexible approach based on nutrition by addition that considers the body's needs in menopause without sliding back into all-or-nothing thinking. Gentle nutrition honors the complexity of being a human in a body that is changing, without making food another thing to get perfect. In *Eat to Thrive During Menopause* (Huber, 2025), I teach women to apply gentle nutrition by adding in foods that nourish both health and satisfaction.

The key is that gentle nutrition comes *after* attunement. Gentle nutrition grows from self-trust. It invites you to experiment with curiosity, not judgment, and to notice what foods fill you up (literally and figuratively), what you enjoy, and what you need more or less of to feel well over time. It's about showing up with care, not control.

REFERENCES

Darpinian, S. (with Sterling, W., & Aggarwal, S.). (2022). *Raising body positive teens: A parent's guide to diet-free living, exercise, and body image*. Jessica Kingsley Publishers.

Huber, J. (2025). *Eat to thrive in menopause: Managing your symptoms with nourishing foods*. Workman Publishing Company.

Kuijer, R. G., & Boyce, J. A. (2014). Chocolate cake. Guilt or celebration? Associations with healthy eating attitudes, perceived behavioural control, intentions and weight-loss. *Appetite*, *74*, 48–54. https://doi.org/10.1016/j.appet.2013.11.013

Boosting Body Confidence in Midlife

Six

One way to think about body image is the picture you have of your body, in your mind's eye, and the way you feel about that picture. It's fair to say we all have a body image. Some of us aren't thinking about it at all, most of us are probably somewhere in the middle, and for some of us, body image takes up a lot of head space, killing confidence in many of our life domains. I don't know anyone who doesn't want to feel better about (or dedicate less head space to) their body, but many of us have no concept of what that would look like.

"Body image is often framed, incorrectly, as a black-and-white issue: Either you feel good about yourself, or you don't. The reality, however, looks more like a spectrum," says Riley Nickols, sport psychologist and eating disorders specialist (Kuzma, 2020, p. 62). On one end of the body image spectrum is body hatred, then there's body tolerance, body acceptance, and then body love at the other end of the spectrum. Nickols says, "Body image shifts in different contexts" (Kuzma, 2020, p. 63). For instance, you might feel confident about your body at work, and insecure about your body in the context of your women's hiking club.

VARIABLES THAT INFLUENCE OUR BODY IMAGE IN MIDLIFE

Everyone in our personal universe influences our body image in positive, negative or neutral ways – family, friends, partners, and co-workers. I notice that when I'm around friends that pour themselves into areas of their lives outside of food preoccupation and body image, it has a positive influence on my own relationship to food and body. Clinical research has shown that negative body talk is contagious and

DOI: 10.4324/9781003632245-9

can hurt friends' body image and reinforce disordered eating (Salk & Engeln-Maddox, 2012).

I can't think about the culture's impact on our body image without thinking about The Fiji Island Study. The bodies that are the most prized in a particular culture are those that the most affluent have. Dr. Anne Becker, anthropologist and psychiatrist at Harvard, oversaw a 1995–1998 study that measured the effect of television on cultural norms. (Television was only catching on in Fiji in 1995. A decade before, even electricity was rare.) Before they had this Western influence through television, there was no prevalence of eating disorders. Fijians had subsistence agriculture at this time, which is where you eat what you grow, and in this type of economy a larger body is typically preferred.

Within three years after Western television was introduced in Fiji (think: Beverly Hills, 90210 and Melrose Place), women and especially teen girls, previously comfortable with their bodies and eating, developed eating disorders at similar rates to their counterparts in the United States. This came from watching shows three hours a week in a communal setting; imagine what media influence has now with an average of six to nine hours a day of screen time! For example, seeing images of the lead female character of Beverly Hills 90210, Kelly Taylor, who was thin and blonde, driving her hot boyfriend around in her convertible sports car and living in a mansion, was just a fraction of the "social storm" television brought to Fijian girls. They saw being blonde and thin was a way to an achieved status in a culture with an ascribed status.

Exposure matters, in my interview with Certified Body Trust® Provider and therapist Dawn Serra, she says, "Many of our preferences – such as those for thinner bodies or taller men – might feel inherent, but they are not, it's conditioning" (Darpinian, 2022). This tracks with the Fiji Island study above: Those studied did not inherently want to be in smaller bodies until they were exposed to the Western images, and started to associate being in a smaller body with an achieved status (Darpinian, 2023).

BACK TO HELEN'S STORY...

Helen learned in therapy that she valued the ability to be more present in her life without the preoccupation that comes with undereating, and constant noise about "what I am going to eat, what I'm not going to eat." She was grateful to no longer reduce her food choices to things like nutrients only, and to bring in aspects including pleasure, celebration, and fun to her relationship with food. She worked hard at the practice of undoing the old conditioning around having her worth come from her body.

During our time together, Helen spent weeks preparing to attend her grandson's highly-anticipated wedding. Of course, it's not a surprise to any of us that there's some pretty intense pressure for a bride to lose weight and be thin for her wedding day. There's particular pressure around the wedding photographs, which will be memorialized for a lifetime. What's not mentioned as much is the pressure the bridal party feels! I have had clients relapse on their eating disorder in preparation to be a bridesmaid. For Helen, attending her grandson's wedding brought up many fears around weight and appearance.

We did many "cope ahead" assignments to prepare Helen for the wedding ahead of time – identifying triggers, rehearsing new emotional responses, and imagining how well the wedding would go, even though she was still grieving the loss of her body as she'd known it. She spent extra time picking out a beautiful dress and shoes, and she achieved being fully present for her grandson's wedding.

To thank Helen, her grandson and her new granddaughter-in-law sent her a framed, poster-sized wedding picture of the whole family. Helen's first reaction to the photo was not positive. She scrutinized herself in the photo, and of course scrutiny breeds dissatisfaction. But as she continues to look at it, her judgmental eye has softened, and she's flooded with sweet memories from that day.

EXPLORATION: DIG, IF YOU WILL, THE PICTURE

If one of the ways you'd like to be different, as it relates to your body, is more body image satisfaction, targeting your response to photos of yourself is a behavior that creates a lot of change. The following exploration will help deal with spiraling body image thoughts after seeing a photo of yourself without letting it take over your day. This even works for Facebook memories!

Brenna O'Malley, RDN and founder of The Wellful provides weight-inclusive nutrition counseling and body image support. She says, "Nobody is going to like every photo of themselves, but we can try to manage the body distress that pictures can bring up" (O'Malley, 2025).

Exploration
by Brenna O'Malley

- Have you ever noticed that you are so focused on what your body looks like in a picture that you don't even see the photo as a whole or the other people in it?
- Does looking at the photo make you doubt the fun you had or even re-write the experience you had on the day the picture was taken?
- Do you have a list of criteria that makes a photo worthy of being printed, posted or shared? Do those rules apply to all people…or only to you?
- It can be helpful to notice how you interact with photos, the pressure you feel around them, and what might feel like auto-pilot when looking at yourself in them.
- How can you reframe your experiences with photos if you notice you are looking at only yourself, or one particular part of your body in a photo?
- See if you can zoom out. What else can you notice? What else was happening while the photo was being taken? Were you celebrating a special day? Were you spending time with people you care about? What does the scenery look like?
- Make a new list of things you notice when looking at a photo. Are your eyes open? Are you smiling? Ask yourself what you want to remember about the day when you see this picture.
- Try the 48-hour rule: Before making any decisions or judgements about deleting a photo, untagging yourself on social media or critiquing your body, wait 48 hours.

WHERE DID YOUR BODY IMAGE COME FROM?

What was the evolution of your body image? What were the messages you received growing up? Are there ways you'd like to feel, think or behave differently regarding your body image? I personally remember the exact messages I received about my body, and you might too.

I like to use a non-body image example to demonstrate the impact of the messages we received in our formative years.

Rocker-turned-neuroscientist Daniel J. Levitin, author of the bestselling book *This is Your Brain on Music*, states that older adults with Alzheimer's Disease can still remember the lyrics to their favorite songs from when they were 14 years old. Why? Because these are the years of self-discovery, and as a consequence, they are emotionally charged. We tend to remember things that have an emotional component; our brain "tags" these memories as something important. (Sidenote: I predict that in 60+ years from now there will be Residential Care Facilities for the elderly full of people singing "Champagne Problems.")

EXPLORATION

What was the evolution of your body image?
What were the messages you received growing up?
Are there ways you'd like to feel, think or behave differently regarding your body image?

DIVERSIFY INTERESTS

Early in my career I went to a talk about self evaluation. The speaker, Dr. Christopher Fairburn, defined self evaluation as, "The way we measure our self worth based on our performance in valued domains." He went on to explain that we are more aware of what matters to us when something in that area of our life goes wrong, than we are when it's going right. He said, "I care about being a good speaker today, but if my wife and I had had a fight before I left the house this morning, that would affect me a lot more than not doing well in this talk today, sorry guys." He was pointing out that his relationship is one of his most valued domains. He might measure his self worth in that domain by how harmonious the relationship is.

Up until then, I hadn't really thought about my own self evaluation. Most of my eggs were in the work basket at that time (before my daughter was born), and even though it's a good basket, having all of your worth come disproportionately from a singular life domain is a slippery slope. If something happens to that basket, it's a total wipe out, it has the potential to destabilize you. Pouring ourselves into other domains is protective against body image dissatisfaction. Nickols calls an over-identification with any one domain a "unidimensional identity." In our interview we talked about how deriving value from your role as a parent, for example, can be healthy, but if you over-identify with your parental identity, you're making a good thing an "ultimate" thing, and a threat like kids going off to college, and no longer needing you in ways they did when they were younger, could cause major distress. Ideally, you want to hold these identities in your mind's eye more abstractly, so that you can have security that this identity is preserved and not entirely dependent on circumstances. For example, telling yourself, "I know I am a mother, even when my daughter isn't with me at the present moment" (Darpinian, 2021).

Having too many eggs in the body image basket is not good. The ways one might measure their self worth in this domain can be harmful: Restricting food, comparing our bodies to other people's, and so on. Expanding one's identity to other areas of life, such as sports, hobbies, or volunteering for an organization that ignites you, allows for different sides of our personalities to be expressed. For example, I can be quite competitive on the tennis court, diving after the ball even if it means I might run into a chain link fence, whereas an intellectually curious side of myself comes out when I'm interviewing a guest on my personal growth podcast. Having our "identity eggs" well distributed in different baskets is protective against a unidimensional identity. If, or when, we feel perceived incompetence or criticism in response to a valued aspect of our identity, we can draw strength from other "eggs."

EXPLORATION: SELF EVALUATION

What are your most valued domains?
How do you measure your self worth based on your performance in this domain?
Do you have too many eggs in one basket?
If so, what would you need to change in order to distribute them more evenly?

THOUGHT HABIT

When we think of "habit," we typically think of a behavior like biting our nails. "Habit of thought" is given less attention. Dr. Dan Tomasulo states, "Your mind will continually make the choices that you've made in the past. We are creatures of habit, but not only habits of behavior – habits of thought and feeling as well. Over time, patterns of thoughts, feelings, and behavior become the default response to a situation" (Tomasulo, 2024).

As a therapist treating body image I often hear, "There is no way I'm ever going to be okay with my bigger body," followed by a feeling of shame or embarrassment. Some clients literally can't remember a time in their lives when they did not have body dissatisfaction. Thoughts are neural firings in the brain, not facts of the universe, but they can certainly feel real. So instead of letting our brain use us, we can choose to be intentional about shifting our gaze to better-feeling thoughts, or use techniques to stop the thoughts once we notice they are happening.

Studies show that driving a taxi in London, with its 25,000 "spaghetti streets" and thousands of landmarks, leads to a larger hippocampus in drivers compared to non-taxi drivers. Learning to navigate these streets is called "The Knowledge," and takes on average three to four years to acquire. It's required to have a license to drive a black cab in London. The hippocampus is the part of the brain associated with spatial intelligence. One could say the hippocampus in the London cabbies is almost "buff." Neurobiologist Howard Eichenbaum of Boston University says he sees it as confirmation of the idea that cognitive exercise produces physical changes in the brain. "The initial findings could have been explained by a correlation, that people with big hippocampi become taxi drivers," he says. "But it turns out it really was the training process that caused the growth in the brain. It shows you can produce profound changes in the brain with training. That's a big deal" (Jabr, 2011).

Whatever we repeat endures, proving that the brain is malleable, even in adulthood. Thought habit, whether negative or positive, shapes the brain to get stronger in those areas. Someone who has practiced negative body image thoughts for as long as they can remember will be able to think those thoughts with little effort. We don't have control over a thought popping up, but we can control how we respond to our thought habits.

The first step to thought habit reversal is awareness.

I just noticed a thought about my body being bigger than it was.

That awareness starts a chain reaction. At first, it won't stop the thoughts from popping up. We only have control over how we respond to the thought, but over time the thought will become more dormant because it won't have as much airtime. The next step, Tomasulo notes, is to take inventory of what you are feeling.

"I'm feeling embarrassed/anxious," and where you are feeling it, e.g. "in my chest/stomach." It doesn't sound like much, but it stops the rumination, and it's providing emotional regulation.

EXPLORATION: THOUGHT HABITS

What thought did you notice?
What are you feeling?
Where are you feeling it?

"FEELING FAT"

"Feeling fat" is illuminated in midlife when bodies are redistributing weight. The idealization of youth and thinness is the problem, not midlife bodies. What's "normal" is size diversity. "Fat" is not a feeling (it's like saying, "I feel hair"). Author Aubrey Gordon, host of Maintenance Phase, says "Fat is not an emotion, it's a body type, it's my body type. It's a phrase we use to mask underlying feelings, so reaching for words that are more precise in describing our emotions can help us get the support we need." Gordon suggests replacement phrases such as, "I'm feeling insecure," or "I'm having a bad body image day," which don't insult others' bodies, or our own (Summers, 2023).

Permitting a whole range of emotions is protective against things like disordered eating and body image dissatisfaction. Learning to hang out in uncomfortable emotions without bringing in a behavior that makes it worse is a DBT skill called Distress Tolerance. This increases the likelihood we won't use maladaptive coping mechanisms to numb ourselves.

FRIENDSHIP WITH BODY

Nickols uses the metaphor of a partnership to describe the two-way relationship we have with our bodies. Nickols extended Timothy Keller's analogy in his book *The Meaning of Marriage*, where there are inevitably going to be seasons in a partnership where we do not like, much less love, our partner. If we behave toward our partner in a manner that is congruent with our feelings (i.e., not liking or loving them), this will likely further and prolong such feelings and corresponding behavior. However, if we can commit to behave toward our partner with respect, even when "You've Lost That Lovin' Feelin," we have a better chance of getting back in alignment with our feelings more quickly. Apply this same principle to your body image.

BODY IMAGE LOSS AND GRIEF

A client of mine, Jessie, sought couple's counseling at the end of her marriage with a man who attempted to control every domain in her life, including her weight. In other words, he asked her to be smaller than her body wanted to be. At their point of attraction, when her self esteem was low, this fit her like a glove. But as she started to evolve, she was able to see his imbalance more clearly. Jessie went on to study weight regulation science as a part of her training in nursing school. After years of study and research, she learned dieting wasn't a valid option because it doesn't work; it's a bandaid fix that leads to food preoccupation. She was no longer willing to have that much room taken up in her head, which she calls "the dieting brain." In her research, she discovered a weight-inclusive medical model committed to doing no harm that resonated with her values as a medical provider. She went on to become a Be Body Positive Facilitator, and provides training for pregnant and parenting teens.

As Jessie moved into midlife and perimenopause, her body started to change, and even though she had a fair amount of body image resilience, she missed feeling like her body was "curvy" and desirable according to societal norms. She felt like her body was now more round. At this point in her journey she had come so far in her body acceptance work that choosing grief over the shame, anxiety, and self loathing that comes from dieting wasn't even a question. Losses such as these are often overlooked.

Katherine Walsh, author of *Grief and Loss*, calls this type of loss "symbolic loss." Says Walsh, "Symbolic loss represents the loss of a role, identity, bodily function, or a relationship. Usually a symbolic loss is not identified as a loss per se, so we may not realize we need to take the time to grieve and to deal with our feelings about it." (Walsh-Burke, 2012, p. 30)

Jessie committed to journaling through her grief to process it, and identified that her *major loss* was "loss of her body as she had known it." The *resulting losses* included the following:

- Perceived loss of desirability to men.
- Loss of respect at the doctor's office, and loss of feeling safe in a medical setting.
- Fear of a lack of credibility at work where she noticed "diet talk" as the norm.
- Loss of a feeling of familiarity when she looked in the mirror.
- A general loss of privilege, especially traveling by airplane. Travel, and the value of adventure, are important to her.

As Jessie's grief started to evolve, she felt ready to do something about it. She started to actively examine the symbolic loss of her self identity being based on having a body that doesn't go through the natural process of aging. In addition, she began to shift from criticizing her body internally to being more discerning and critical of societal norms that define women's worthiness by their body shape, size, and youth. She started to have more clarity of mind, and did writing with prompts like; "Why am I examining my body through the male gaze?", "Where am I getting this?", and "Who says I have the wrong body?"

Grieving the loss of body as you've known it, or how you'd hoped it would be, is not a one-time deal. As her therapist, I knew that grief doesn't have an end, but instead offers a doorway of growth to walk through, again and again. Dr. Linda Shanti, grief and body image expert says, "Unlike what we used to think with stage models of grief, such as Kubler Ross's 5 Stages, we now know that grief is a nonlinear process that is never done, but an ongoing opportunity to grow, learn, and become a different person."

Jessie uses the mantra, "This is healing pain and I will grow from it," to help reduce suffering, as well as journaling to reframe unpleasant events related to her body image. Journaling has been shown to regulate emotion with benefits that last at least a month (Kam et al., 2024).

EXPLORATION: BODY IMAGE GRIEF

What are the "Major Loss" and "Resulting Losses" you've experienced with regards to your body?

Major Loss____________________

Resulting Losses_________________

REFERENCES

Darpinian, S. (2021, February 24). Cultivating mental and physical health in athletes. *Therapy Rocks!* https://audioboom.com/posts/7809114-cultivating-mental-and-physical-health-in-athletes

Darpinian, S. (2022, August 1). Let's talk about sex... *Therapy Rocks!* https://audioboom.com/posts/8130249-let-s-talk-about-sex

Darpinian, S. (2023, February 13). From the fiji islands to facebook: The impact of westernized media on the island of fiji. *Therapy Rocks!* https://audioboom.com/posts/8246958-from-the-fiji-islands-to-facebook-the-impact-of-westernized-media-on-the-island-of-fiji

Jabr, F. (2011, December 8). Cache cab: Taxi drivers' brains grow to navigate london's streets. *Scientific American*. https://www.scientificamerican.com/article/london-taxi-memory/

Kam, J. W. Y., Wan-Sai-Cheong, L., Zuk, A. A. O., Mehta, A., Dixon, M. L., & Gross, J. J. (2024). A brief reappraisal intervention leads to durable affective benefits. *Emotion (Washington, D.C.)*, 24(7), 1676–1688. https://doi.org/10.1037/emo0001391

Kuzma, C. (2020, July 14). What is healthy body image, anyways? *Women's Running*. https://www.womensrunning.com/health/wellness/healthy-body-image-defined/

O'Malley, B. (2025). *Home*. The Wellful. https://thewellful.com/

Salk, R. H., & Engeln-Maddox, R. (2012). Fat talk among college women is both contagious and harmful. *Sex Roles*, 66(9–10), 636–645. https://doi.org/10.1007/s11199-011-0050-1

Summers, J. (2023, January 9). Author Aubrey Gordon wants to change the way you think—And talk—About fat people. *NPR*. https://www.npr.org/2023/01/09/1147909132/author-aubrey-gordon-wants-to-change-the-way-you-think-and-talk-about-fat-people

Tomasulo, D. (2024, November 9). *How the science of hope can change negative habits into positivity*. DAN TOMASULO. https://www.dantomasulo.com/blog/how-the-science-of-hope-can-change-negative-habits-into-positivity

Walsh-Burke, K. (2012). *Grief and loss: Theories and skills for the helping professions* (2nd ed.). Pearson.

Movement in Midlife

Seven

Women in midlife don't often have a lot of free time for exercise. I just talked to my friend Luzi about it and she said, "I have two teenagers in the house, I run a preschool that's essentially an urban farm populated with two-five year olds, potbelly pigs, bunnies, guinea pigs and cats plus an occasional rat." She went on to say that she'd rather spend her free time doing her work around personal growth than physical fitness. She's content with the daily activity she gets running a preschool, and her routine of walking the dogs after a long day at work. She told me, "I feel like I'd just be exercising so that I could be desired by someone, and that doesn't feel like the right reason. The desire to move should come from inside of me."

It's unfortunate that our culture puts an emphasis on exercising as a way to change the shape of our body (code for being thin). While exercise is very important to health, it's not likely to lead to long-term weight loss (Bacon & Aphramor, 2014). Studies show that exercising for external reasons is not sustainable, not to mention it can feel unenjoyable. The goal is to move for internal reasons (if moving more is something you'd like to do). This makes movement more sustainable in the long run.

In this chapter we'll talk about the benefits of exercising in a manner that supports your stage of life, interests, and connectedness to others. And yes, walking the dog counts!

MOVEMENT MAKES US HAPPY

You've heard that exercise can increase human happiness, but do you know why? I interviewed Dr. Kelly McGonigal, health psychologist and lecturer at Stanford University, author of *The Joy of Movement*.

DOI: 10.4324/9781003632245-10

Says McGonigal, "Regular activity changes your brain in ways that make you enjoy it and want to do it more, particularly if it is done in combination with other things that activate the reward system. For some people that's music, for others it's exercising in nature, some value competition, and for some the reward is connectedness with other people."

McGonigal says there are a couple of prerequisites to activating this reward system: One is that it needs to be at least twenty minutes of movement that gets your heart rate up at least a little bit, and the other is that your brain needs to interpret it as an activity that has meaning to you. This tracks with my friend's story in the beginning of this chapter: Her daily walks are combined with two dogs she's deeply bonded to, walking them is as meaningful to her for their well-being as it is her own. She walks them for over twenty minutes (without thinking about it) in the hills of the East Bay, California, which naturally leads to the exertion her brain needs to activate the reward system. For her this is rewarding in a way a treadmill would not be.

Says McGonigal, "You can't be active without having an increase in dopamine, the brain chemical that drives the reward system and positive motivation, because dopamine is the key neurotransmitter of physical movement. Also, through most forms of movement you will get increases in brain chemicals like endocannabinoids, endorphins and sometimes oxytocin and serotonin." She explains that when you experience a high or reward from activity, it's a very different type of high than you would get from a type of drug that would cause a destructive dependence. Exercise seems to be a reward that rewards you while you do it and it sensitizes your brain to other pleasures, so that sunsets are more beautiful, friends' jokes are funnier, and reading a book is more interesting. This is also why exercise is very supportive for people who are depressed, grieving, or recovering from addiction; in all of these cases the reward system is blunted. In its way, exercise is a highly effective antidepressant (Darpinian, 2021a).

We also talked about how some people are not inclined to move because they have not found the right exercise. Look for communities and organizations that support you with whatever your needs are, whether it's your age, starting a physical activity for the first time, or looking for a Master's exercise group of some kind. Some Master's swim groups, for example, are very competitive and regularly participate in swim meets, while others are not competitive at all and simply have daily workouts to follow, but with no consequences if you opt to do your own workout. For any Master's exercise group, the biggest reward is being part of a community of people that love exercising or playing a sport with one another.

Exercise avoidance can also be related to mental, physical, and cognitive challenges. If that's the case, McGonigal suggests Adaptive Fitness, an online resource that embodies inclusivity and support, making fitness accessible to most (*Adaptive Fitness*, 2025). There is no expiration date, you can start at any age, even if you've identified yourself as someone who doesn't like to exercise, McGonigal states that it takes about six weeks of a particular movement, for the changes to occur in the brain.

LOVE FORTY

"What's the score?"

"Did you just serve or did I?"

Ah, playing tennis in midlife and beyond with brain fog. When one tennis partner is in perimenopause, and the other is postmenopausal, you might want to keep the score using the honor system.

Elia played lots of sports growing up. She was a good skier, but really fell in love with snowboarding as a young adult. She said, "It feels like surfing down a mountain." Outside of ski season, she had a pattern of getting a gym membership that would last an average of six months, but the lack of reward she got from the stationary machines at the gym made it hard to stay in the habit of moving. Elia stopped snowboarding when she had kids, and when they grew older and she got back into snowboarding, she felt she was holding back because she was more concerned about potential injuries in midlife. She did have a committed yoga practice up until the pandemic, when she had to leave her yoga studio and shift gears to online classes at home – this didn't last long.

At age 46, friends encouraged her to try tennis for the first time. Still in COVID lockdown, outdoor tennis courts seemed like the perfect destination. Tennis courts at parks turned into a membership at a gym that actually lasted this time. Playing singles tennis led to the tennis team and opened her world up to new people. When asked what she loves about tennis, Elia, now 49, said, "I think one of the things I like about tennis is that I have to do it with someone, which makes me get out of the house and do it. Otherwise I get busy or lazy and just want to stay home. That's why I was able to stick with yoga when I was doing it with friends before COVID. I guess I'm a social exerciser." Elia also likes that she can see improvements in her game over time as she continues to learn new techniques. During tennis season she plays up to four days a week, and says she never gets burnt out, because it feels more like a hobby than exercise.

CONNIE ON CLIMBING

Physical activity that takes place in a natural environment is called "green exercise." Unlike a runner's high, the mind-altering effects of green exercise kick in almost immediately (McGonigal, 2019). Whether your exercise takes place indoors or outdoors in nature, physical activity can be an act of self-care, even self-preservation. I asked Connie Sobczak, co-founder of The Body Positive and author of *Embody*, to explain how climbing strengthened her self trust and helped her reframe her aging body.

> Nature has healed me in many ways throughout my life. For more than sixty years, I have been going to a very special mountain lake every summer. I started rock climbing there at the age of 12 with a friend of mine. We free climbed because we never thought of doing it another way. What I learned from climbing was to trust my body. If I'd move a hand or a foot, and not do it right, I could fall and die, so I learned to deeply trust myself. The lessons I learned on the mountain came home with me. I realized that when I was in nature, on granite, in trees, in the water, I felt like I was a part of something bigger than myself. As my body's aged, I've had so much fun seeing it as a natural wonder. I have a favorite tree on the mountain that I visit at the lake every summer. I put my hands on the tree, and they look like the bark as they've gotten wrinkly, rough, and marked. They become part of the tree, and I can see their incredible beauty. Seeing my aging body as a natural wonder is not always the first thing I see. My practice, though, when I do look at an aging part of my body and say, "Eww!" is to recognize that it's the conditioned response that was planted in my brain from a very early age – the

cultural messaging that *this* is beauty, and *this* is not. My practice is to hear the conditioned message, and then take time with it and reframe it.

(Darpinian, 2021b)

EXPLORATION

What's your conditioned response when you first see your aging body while exercising?
Can you craft a new response?

HABIT FORMATION AROUND MOVEMENT

Habit is a word we use all the time. Dr. Joanna Steinglass, Professor of Psychiatry in the Columbia Center for Eating Disorders, says when we are using the word "habit" from a neuroscience perspective, it's important to highlight that particular definition, "Habits are behaviors that are learned, they are not innate like "reflexes" or something we are born with, and they develop over time. As you learn to do the same thing in the same setting, over and over again, eventually it gets stamped in, and shifts to a more entrenched part of the brain" (Darpinian, 2020).

Up until fairly recently, I was out of the habit of strength training. I had negative associations with this particular type of exercise. It felt too hard and I seemed to get injured too often, in other words, there wasn't enough of a "reward" for me to repeat the behavior. In our interview together, Steinglass used animal literature around habit, "If you have a rat, and you put it in a cage, and you train it to press a lever to get a reward, it eventually learns, "if I press this lever I get a reward." And if the rat does this over and over and over again, at some point the rat will continue to press the lever even if the reward is taken away." Steinglass says this is when it's considered to be a habit because the behavior persists despite the diminished reward. In other words, behaviors become habitual when they are rewarding (at least at the beginning) and are done multiple times.

If you are looking to increase your habit of exercise, in this case strength training, consider using a research-based intervention on the latest neuroscience of habit from Colombia's team.

In my midlife and menopause studies it became clearer that incorporating strength training into my exercise routine was a "health behavior" worth improving, so I decided to give it another try. I signed up for a "live" class at my gym. Crystal, the instructor, holds certifications in a variety of group fitness formats from HIIT cardio to strength training to mobility training. She starts class by letting new members know what the class is, to help them feel comfortable coming to a class for the first time. She says, "It can be intimidating to walk into a class where everyone seems to already know each other, as well as what to do. It's also important to remind regular members why they are here." The class is focused on mobility, stability, balance, functional strength, and flexibility – areas she says, "most people don't tend to focus on, or feel is necessary to, but it is necessary, especially as we get older, to teach unilateral movements (working one side of the body at a time) to help improve any imbalances we have."

The key to getting started is to first pick a time that you could repeat regularly. The class I signed up for is 10:30 a.m. on Sundays. This is an easy time of the morning for me to be somewhere, which matters, because if the class was at 6:30 a.m., it would be too painful for me to sustain my attendance.

Next, take a good look at your routine. Look for the moment in the sequence of events in which it's easiest to take a different path. For example, if I wake up by 7:30 a.m. on a Sunday, I can enjoy a couple hours of relaxing with a cup of coffee and writing in my journal. By the time 9:30 rolls around, I'm ready to switch gears and head to class. If I slept until 8:30, I might not go, because I'd be missing my chill time. Only you know your routine and the timing that's most likely to create a sustainable path for you.

Second, set up external cues in your environment while initiating your new habit. For example, I put my purple yoga mat right by my bedroom door so it's the first thing I see when I wake up on Sunday morning.

Finally, make sure you pay attention to what you enjoy about the new routine. I enjoy getting to class early so I can chat with my new acquaintances while waiting for class to start. I love the way I feel strong in my body after class. Research has shown that exercise can improve a person's body image, regardless of any actual change in their body. One study showed that just 30 minutes of physical activity had a significant positive effect on women's body image (Salci & Martin Ginis, 2017).

I no longer get injured now that Crystal watches my form and teaches the class how to properly lift weights. She says, "The better your form, the better your results, and lifting with good form also keeps you from getting injured. Using modifications or lower intensity movements when needed is essential too. If I teach different options and encourage everyone to use them without feeling like they aren't strong enough, it hopefully gets people to keep moving while listening to their bodies. If people leave feeling good physically and mentally, strong, accomplished, less stressed, and glad they came, it makes it a routine they want to stick to."

B. Timothy Walsh of the Columbia Center for Eating Disorders notes that once behaviors become linked together into a routine, and once the chain of action is initiated, the rest follows with little mental effort. Creating a new habit is called "habit formation." Habit formation is the process by which new behaviors become automatic (Glasofer & Steinglass, 2016). If you feel inclined to grab your yoga mat at 10:00 on a Sunday morning to head to class with Crystal, you've acquired a habit.

IS YOUR MOVEMENT NUTRITIONALLY SUPPORTED?

In Chapter One, we talked about the most common first sign of early perimenopause being cycle irregularity. Dr. Nanette Sontoro says, "If it looks like a duck, and walks like a duck, you don't need a test to determine perimenopause if you are in the right age group" (*Menopause Step by Step | Professional Resources*, 2025). But on occasion, it looks like a duck, walks like a duck, but is in fact, a rabbit. It takes me back to the days of reading Amy Krouse Rosenthal's thought-provoking children's book *Duck! Rabbit!* that uses the age-old optical illusion: Is it a duck or a rabbit? Depends on how you look at it! As an eating disorder therapist, I'm accustomed to clients at all stages of life having an interruption in their menstrual pattern that is frequently overlooked by healthcare professionals.

If a woman has lost her period at the median age of perimenopause or younger, and it's in the presence of underfueling (at any weight, not just low weight) or over-exercising, it could be both a duck and a rabbit. I'm not going to assume she is entering the menopause transition until I am certain she is weight restored and eating and exercising in a balanced manner, as determined by a multidisciplinary team specialized in eating disorders: Physician, mental health provider, and dietician. Board-Certified Sports Dietitian (CSSD) Wendy Sterling says, "Your menstrual cycle can serve as a 'check engine light' for your body. Your menstrual cycle might be sending you a message that you need to slow down, take a rest day, add an extra snack." If the body doesn't have enough fuel, it is not going to expend precious energy on non-essential things like menstruation. If it's determined that the loss of cycle is the byproduct of underfueling, taking into consideration an individual's energy needs, including their exercise, this is called Relative Energy Deficiency in Sport (REDs).

RELATIVE ENERGY DEFICIENCY IN SPORT

by Riley Nickols, PhD, CEDS-C

Dr. Riley Nickols, founder of Mind Body Endurance, a practice of specialized services for those competing in sport, as well as treatment for eating disorders in sport, says that in the 1990s, the American College of Sports Medicine (ACSM) developed the Female Athlete Triad (Otis et al., 1997), comprising three conditions: Low bone mineral density, functional hypothalamic amenorrhea, and low energy availability (LEA). In 2014, the International Olympic Committee (IOC) expanded upon the Female Athlete Triad to acknowledge that energy deficiency impacts all athletes, not just females, and to broaden the scope of the syndrome beyond just menstrual dysfunction and bone health. They replaced the Female Athlete Triad with Relative Energy Deficiency in Sport (REDs) (Mountjoy et al., 2014). This new definition explains the far-reaching implications, including effects on the brain and body, that can occur when the body is in a state of LEA for a prolonged period of time.

Says Nickols:

> Exercise has long been shown to reduce stress hormones while also improving mood, cognitive functioning, and sleep quality. The benefits of exercise will not be maximized unless there is enough nutritional intake to support the increased energy demands of exercise. Additionally,

sufficient nutrition in the context of exercise is important to facilitate the body's recovery and prevent injuries. Exercise that is enjoyable and nutritionally supported can best allow you to experience enhanced mood and sleep, both of which can be disrupted in the menopause transition.

IS IT PERIMENOPAUSE OR RELATIVE ENERGY DEFICIENCY IN SPORT?

by Val Schonberg, RD, CSSD, Menopause Certified Practitioner (MSCP)

Symptoms like irregular or absent periods, mood changes, fatigue, inability to lose weight, low bone density, sleep disturbances, and decreased performance are often linked to perimenopause (Monteleone et al., 2018). But every one of these signs can also point to Relative Energy Deficiency in Sport (REDs), making an accurate diagnosis in middle-aged active women difficult (Mountjoy et al., 2023).

While perimenopause is a reasonable consideration – especially since natural menopause can begin as early as 45 – focusing solely on menopause can delay recognition of an underlying energy imbalance. If REDs is the root cause, behavioral changes to restore energy balance are essential for resuming normal menstrual function and preventing long-term health risks. If perimenopause or early menopause is confirmed, menopause hormone therapy (MHT) may be beneficial. In both cases, addressing nutrient needs, such as low iron, calcium, vitamin D, and carbohydrates, is critical for supporting physical and mental health – as well as future training.

DIAGNOSTIC CONSIDERATIONS

Hormone testing is commonly suggested, but it's often unreliable during perimenopause due to natural fluctuations. For this reason, major menopause and endocrine societies do not recommend routine hormone testing to assess menopausal status (Stuenkel, 2024). Gynecologists may recommend testing for women under 45 with over four months of amenorrhea to rule out other causes of amenorrhea, such as pregnancy or early menopause (ESHRE, ASRM, CREWHIRL and IMS Guideline Group on POI et al., 2024). For example, follicle-stimulating hormone (FSH) is a test that, when it is elevated, indicates menopause.

Complicating matters, functional hypothalamic amenorrhea (FHA) – one of the signs of REDs – can appear to be perimenopause in middle-aged active women. FHA is triggered by stressors including undernutrition, overtraining, and psychological strain, which disrupt ovulation and lower estrogen.

Diagnosing REDs presents its own challenges. Accurate measurement of energy availability requires data on fat-free mass, dietary intake, and energy expenditure through exercise – all of which are prone to measurement errors and variability in the methods used to estimate energy availability (Burke et al., 2018).

A comprehensive REDs assessment is best done by a multidisciplinary team including physicians, dietitians, and mental health professionals. This includes a detailed medical history, physical exam, and lab work, along with a review of training, menstrual history, and performance concerns. Sports dietitians play a key role by evaluating dietary habits, weight history, and exercise training, including the type, frequency, intensity of activity, and any recent changes in their exercise patterns.

Research shows that low energy availability – especially with inadequate carbohydrate intake – negatively affects bone health, immunity, and iron status. In today's weight-focused culture, the issue is amplified by the emphasis on high-protein diets, which further reduce carbohydrate availability.

NUTRITIONAL REHABILITATION

Nutritional rehabilitation is required to reverse REDs. Athletes often benefit from individualized meal planning that prioritizes foods to support physiological health and reintroduces restricted foods, such as carbohydrates, back into their diet. Understandably, many midlife women are hesitant to eat more due to fear of weight gain.

Sports dietitians play a key role by partnering with women to explain the purpose behind dietary changes that support long-term health and well-being, while dispelling common myths about nutrition, weight, and performance. Shifting the focus from weight to fueling for health and healing helps rebuild trust in the body. Often, body image work and psychological support are essential parts of the recovery process.

UNPACKING MISINFORMATION

Letting go of food rules and navigating pervasive misinformation isn't easy. Many midlife female athletes are told that eating more protein and lifting heavy weights will resolve their weight concerns by gaining muscle and losing fat. Others hear that they simply need to "gain weight" to recover from REDs, which triggers fear and resistance. While these messages can be well-meaning, they oversimplify a far more complex issue.

The truth is no one can define a biologically optimal weight or body composition for an individual woman – especially during midlife and the menopause transition. While studies may offer averages about weight at this stage of life, women want to know what will happen to *them*. That level of insight can only come from personalized care and a realistic, sustainable nutrition plan.

THE BIGGER PICTURE

Distinguishing between REDs and perimenopause isn't easy. Many women lack access to specialized care and general practitioners may not have the time, training, or awareness to recognize the signs of low energy availability. Furthermore, reliance on weight as a marker of health often leads to misdiagnosis or missed opportunities for intervention.

Regardless of body size, it's essential to look beyond menopause when evaluating disruptive symptoms in active women. Missing REDs not only delays recovery, but it can also lead to irreversible bone loss and long-term health consequences. However, recognizing and treating low energy availability is key to relieving symptoms, protecting long-term health, and helping women rediscover lasting joy in their sport.

THE ROLE OF PELVIC HEALTH THERAPY IN MIDLIFE AND BEYOND

by Anietie Ukpe-Wallace, PT, DPT

Anietie Ukpe-Wallace is a board-certified physical therapist who specializes in pelvic health. She says, "Most people don't give much thought or consideration to pelvic health unless they are pregnant or when something is wrong." But we can't talk about movement in midlife without also talking about pelvic health.

The pelvis is like the rudder of a ship, or to put it another way, the keystone for a building; it provides both the direction and the foundation for our bodies. Think about it this way: When you sprain your ankle, you will notice that as you are recovering from that injury, your gait will dramatically change, creating changes from your feet all the way up through your spine. You may bear less weight on that leg or walk in a different way to avoid going into pain. All of this will then affect the mobility of your pelvis and spine, as well as how you move about in the world. Increasing body literacy, as it relates to pelvic health in midlife and beyond, is crucial to preserving your relationship to movement/exercise. Pelvic floor muscle training (PFMT) is defined as an exercise program aimed to increase muscle strength, endurance, power, flexibility, and relaxation of the pelvic floor muscles (PFM) (Derbyshire, 2021).

Hormonal changes that can have such a huge impact when we enter the perimenopause and menopause space also have an impact on our pelvic health. The fluctuations in estrogen and decline of progesterone and testosterone can affect our ability to maintain optimal bladder, bowel and sexual health, due to the loss of elasticity and lubrication in the tissues of the pelvic bowl. This is Genitourinary Syndrome of Menopause (GSM). GSM can affect the ability for the sphincter muscles around the urethra to contract as needed to prevent leakage or for sufficient lubrication that is needed for vaginal insertion with intercourse. In Chapter One, we considered a hormonal option for treating GSM – topical local estrogen therapy in the vagina and vulvar region. The frontline non hormonal treatment is pelvic floor therapy, which can be easily combined with hormonal treatment (Association, 2025).

Kegels are the go-to exercise for most women with these symptoms, and the most "prescribed" by many medical establishments, but unfortunately most women are doing Kegels incorrectly by recruiting the wrong muscles. When we know how to optimally engage these Kegel muscles it can be a lot easier to then integrate them into our regular exercises and strength training routine. Ideally, these muscles need to do much more than just squeeze, they need the ability to lift as well. The coordination of the breathing diaphragm, the deep core muscles, and the PFM all work in concert with each other to ensure a strong and resilient pelvic bowl.

To prescribe an exercise for the pelvic floor, such as a Kegels, in a book format would not be wise, given that there's no way to ensure it is being done correctly. However, below is an experiential technique that's the foundation for learning how to recruit pelvic bowl muscles.

Start by inserting a finger into the vagina to help you feel the contraction and relaxation of your muscles. If you prefer not to do that, placing a finger on your perineum (the space between your vaginal opening and anus) can work just as well. Take a deep breath in through your nose and you should feel for downward movement of your pelvic bowl. When you exhale gently, you should feel a natural recoil of your pelvic bowl muscles drawing back up to their original position. This may be subtle for some and for others, they feel a lot or nothing at all. All of this is good information.

Now try to do this again and as you exhale, imagine that you are blowing out through a straw or blowing up a balloon. As you do this, you should feel two things: Even more squeezing occurring around your finger or at the perineum as well as a "drawing up" movement of your finger as if being sucked upwards. This is the work of the deep core and breathing diaphragm helping to hold the container and provide support for your pelvic bowl.

Think of your pelvic bowl like a trampoline. The jumping mat consists of the three layers of pelvic muscles, the metal frame is the bony structure and the springs are the tendons and ligaments that connect the layers of muscles to the bony pelvis. When those muscles are at rest, there is an underlying amount of tension or holding that is happening; this is what our pelvic bowl muscles are doing all day, every day as they manage the different pressures in our body during exercise, when we are standing or even when we sneeze! When someone jumps on the trampoline, noticeable lengthening occurs, but still some percentage of tension is there. When we have a bowel movement, the lengthening is just enough so that we don't have our insides fall out every time we poop and so that our pelvic bowl muscles have the ability to return back to their original form.

When we are doing a Kegel or other form of strengthening our pelvic bowl, not only are we creating better support for our pelvic organs, but we are also encouraging better movement for those muscles that connect to our pelvis, hips, and spine. This is especially important in midlife and beyond. When the pelvic bowl muscles are constantly lengthening and contracting and having to work, whether it is with our own bodyweight or weights like dumbbells or kettlebells, the muscles are pulling on the bony structure of the pelvis via the tendons, causing not just movement of the joints in our hips and pelvis but also encouraging more bone tissue growth thus increasing our bone density. When we create a healthy amount of tone in our pelvic bowl, we can positively influence the health of our hips and spine.

Strengthening our pelvic bowl muscles can counter the effects of GSM. In a systematic review conducted in 2024, researchers looked at the use of Kegels and pelvic floor muscle (PFM) training and their impact on quality of life for postmenopausal women with GSM. What they found is that Kegels significantly improved urinary symptom-related health-related quality of life in postmenopausal women, thus improving urinary leakage due to strengthening of the pelvic floor muscles, making those muscles that sit under the uterus and bladder stronger and preventing sagging into the vagina (Nguyen et al., 2024).

The study also concluded that although Kegels are great for PFM and that they play a role in sexual function, they do not solely affect sexual symptoms of GSM as there are many other interpersonal, sociocultural, and hormonal impacts. In patients with GSM and psychosocial and/or sexual health concerns, referring to a sex therapist in addition to a pelvic floor physical therapist can be helpful.

WHERE CAN I GO FOR HELP?

Despite the potentially disruptive nature of GSM, only about half of individuals with GSM symptoms report discussing their symptoms with their doctors, and of those who did, most said the doctor did not initiate the conversation. Lauren Streicher, MD, MSCP, who spoke on sexual function at The Menopause Society's 2024 Annual Meeting said, "Ideally, a clinician would be asking, 'Are you happy with your sexual function?'" (Streicher, 2024). The good news is that there is help beyond what you may receive when you go to your primary care doctor. Many pelvic health therapists are trained to address the vulvovaginal conditions that can occur in perimenopause and menopause. When working with a clinician who will take the time to listen to your concerns, you can feel stronger in your body, understand your symptoms, and learn to navigate the tumultuous changes occurring in your body. If you are experiencing vaginal, urinary, or sexual symptoms, let your doctor know. It's time to start normalizing these conversations.

In patients with GSM and pelvic floor dysfunction, clinicians may refer to a physical therapist specializing in pelvic floor conditions. If your doctor does not provide you with a referral, there are a number of online directories of local pelvic health therapists. If you live in an area where there are no pelvic health therapists nearby, many offer a telehealth option, which is a great way to still get the care you need, virtually. See Resources at the end of this book.

REFERENCES

Adaptive Fitness. (2025). Special Strong. https://adaptivefitness.com/

Association, A. U. (2025, April 28). *American urological association releases new guideline on genitourinary syndrome of menopause*. GlobeNewswire News Room. https://www.globenewswire.com/news-release/2025/04/28/3069422/0/en/American-Urological-Association-Releases-New-Guideline-on-Genitourinary-Syndrome-of-Menopause.html

Bacon, L., & Aphramor, L. (2014). *Body respect:What conventional health books get wrong, leave out, and just plain fail to understand about weight*. BenBella Books, Inc.

Burke, L. M., Lundy, B., Fahrenholtz, I. L., & Melin, A. K. (2018). Pitfalls of conducting and interpreting estimates of energy availability in free-living athletes. *International Journal of Sport Nutrition and Exercise Metabolism*, 28(4), 350–363. https://doi.org/10.1123/ijsnem.2018-0142

Darpinian, S. (2020, August 7). *Disrupting habits that don't help*. Therapy Rocks! https://audioboom.com/posts/7651840-disrupting-habits-that-don-t-help

Darpinian, S. (2021a, July 3). *The joy of movement*. Therapy Rocks! https://audioboom.com/posts/7898299-the-joy-of-movement

Darpinian, S. (2021b, November 9). *The art of aging*. Therapy Rocks! https://audioboom.com/posts/7975329-the-art-of-aging

Derbyshire, M. (2021, March 15). *Pelvic floor muscle training as a treatment for genitourinary syndrome of menopause*. International Menopause Society. https://www.imsociety.org/2021/03/15/pelvic-floor-muscle-training-as-a-treatment-for-genitourinary-syndrome-of-menopause/

ESHRE, ASRM, CREWHIRL and IMS Guideline Group on POI, Panay, N., Anderson, R. A., Bennie, A., Cedars, M., Davies, M., Ee, C., Gravholt, C. H., Kalantaridou, S., Kallen, A., Kim, K. Q., Misrahi, M., Mousa, A., Nappi, R. E., Rocca, W. A., Ruan, X., Teede, H., Vermeulen, N., Vogt, E., & Vincent, A. J. (2024). Evidence-based guideline: Premature ovarian insufficiency. *Climacteric: The Journal of the International Menopause Society*, 27(6), 510–520. https://doi.org/10.1080/13697137.2024.2423213

Glasofer, D. R., & Steinglass, J. (2016). Disrupting the habits of anorexia. *Scientific American Mind*, 27(5), 27–29. https://doi.org/10.1038/scientificamericanmind0916-27

McGonigal, K. (2019). *The joy of movement: How exercise helps us find happiness, hope, connection, and courage*. Penguin Publishing Group.

Menopause Step by Step | Professional Resources. (2025). The Menopause Society. https://menopause.org/professional-resources/step-by-step

Monteleone, P., Mascagni, G., Giannini, A., et al. (2018). Symptoms of menopause – global prevalence, physiology and implications. *Nat Rev Endocrinol*, 14(4), 199–215.

Mountjoy, M., Sundgot-Borgen, J., Burke, L., Carter, S., Constantini, N., Lebrun, C., Meyer, N., Sherman, R., Steffen, K., Budgett, R., & Ljungqvist, A. (2014). The ioc consensus statement: Beyond the female athlete triad—relative energy deficiency in sport (Red-s). *British Journal of Sports Medicine*, 48(7), 491–497. https://doi.org/10.1136/bjsports-2014-093502

Mountjoy, M., Ackerman, K. E., Bailey, D. M., Burke, L. M., Constantini, N., Hackney, A. C., Heikura, I. A., Melin, A., Pensgaard, A. M., Stellingwerff, T., Sundgot-Borgen, J. K., Torstveit, M. K., Jacobsen, A. U., Verhagen, E., Budgett, R., Engebretsen, L., & Erdener, U. (2023). 2023 International Olympic Committee's (IOC) consensus statement on Relative Energy Deficiency in Sport (REDs). *British Journal of Sports Medicine*, 57(17), 1073–1097. https://doi.org/10.1136/bjsports-2023-106994

Nguyen, T. T. B., Hsu, Y.-Y., & Sari, Y. P. (2024). The effect of pelvic floor muscle training on health-related quality of life in postmenopausal women with genitourinary syndrome: A systematic review and meta-analysis. *Journal of Nursing Research*, 32(1), e316. https://doi.org/10.1097/jnr.0000000000000597

Otis, C. L., Drinkwater, B., Johnson, M., Loucks, A., & Wilmore, J. (1997). Acsm position stand: The female athlete triad. *Medicine & Science in Sports & Exercise*, 29(5), i–ix. https://doi.org/10.1097/00005768-199705000-00037

Salci, L. E., & Martin Ginis, K. A. (2017). Acute effects of exercise on women with pre-existing body image concerns: A test of potential mediators. *Psychology of Sport and Exercise*, 31, 113–122. https://doi.org/10.1016/j.psychsport.2017.04.001

Streicher, L. (2024, September 10). *Sexual function 101*. Menopause Society Annual Meeting. https://watch.ondemand.org/player/30984/86480/sessions-630

Stuenkel, C. A. (2024). What is menopause? *Menopause*, 31(9), 837–838. https://doi.org/10.1097/GME.0000000000002416

PART 4
Enhancing Midlife

The Power of Midlife Friendships

Eight

We have so much diet culture messaging coming our way that it's easy to feel like our health can be reduced to the food we eat and what we weigh. In actuality, neither are true. You could never look at someone and determine their health. Our health is more like a 1,000 piece puzzle with many tiny little components.

What often gets left out of our health equation is our friendships. The Harvard Study of Adult Development, the longest running study on living a longer and more satisfying life, found that close friendships, more than money, fame, or even cholesterol levels, are connected to keeping people happy and healthy in the long term. Psychiatrist Robert Waldinger, the current director of the 75-year-old study on adult development said in his TED Talk, "Good relationships keep us happier and healthier. Period. Social connections are really good for us, and loneliness kills. People who are more socially connected to family, to friends, and community are happier, they're physically healthier, and they live longer than people who are more isolated than they want to be from others" (Waldinger, 2015).

Waldinger goes on to say that It's not the number of friends but the quality of the friendships. If we think back to the COVID-19 pandemic, we saw people finding creative ways to stay connected to their friends through Netflix movie nights, FaceTime calls, and drive-by birthday parties. Friendships buffer our stress response; they help us handle our stress. Dr. Elizabeth Laugeson, author of *The Science of Making Friends* and founder of PEERS Clinic at UCLA says, "Most people have one or two close friends. People with close friendships are less likely to be depressed or anxious, have better self esteem and they are more independent."

DOI: 10.4324/9781003632245-12

Some people have close friends that they've had most of their lives. It's unique to have someone that we have all of that shared history with, especially if you've been able to "grow" together. But sometimes we're encouraged to hang onto old friendships for the wrong reasons, even though we may no longer be bringing out the best in each other. Laugeson says these are people who are "committed" to the history of the friendship. The fact is that we're not the same as we were when we first met our lifelong friends. We can still value these friendships for the history of them, even if we decide to go our separate ways.

A motto at the UCLA PEERS Clinic is, "Friendship is a choice, and people change, so friendships change." Says Laugeson, "Normalizing this is the first step. It starts the thought process. Forcing friendships doesn't work, and it certainly doesn't lead to healthy relationships."

I remember being in middle school and high school and spending hours upon hours with my closest friends. We'd listen to music together, watch soap operas, and try on different identities as we started to figure out who we were. At that age, we didn't realize there wasn't going to be another time in life like that, given that our priorities would naturally change as we grew older. As adults we don't have the same time to spend with our friends, so quality time becomes more important than quantity.

Midlife marks an interesting time for existing friendships and making new friends. Tending to our existing friendships and making new friends tends to be on the backburner – we're focused on our careers and our kids – often, for ease, making friends with the parents of our kid's friends. As I'm writing this, I'm realizing I need to prioritize more "date nights" with these friends so we'll have a relationship to fall back on when the kids fly the nest. (This is a topic typically reserved for romantic relationships.) Break-ups are reserved for romantic relationships too, and no one discusses the grief associated with breaking up with a friend or changing our relationship with them. For example, a best friendship might morph into more of a regular friendship, or even just a cordial acquaintanceship. Our friendships deserve more attention than we often give them, especially since they are so linked to happiness throughout our lifespan.

Friends are at different stages in midlife: Some of us are raising kids in elementary school, some are empty nesters or grandparents, some are at the top of their game in their career, and some are retired.

Midlife circumstances vary, but if you are reading this book it's possible you no longer have the advantage of making friends through your kids' playdates (if having kids was something you chose to do) or through your work.

Midlife is another time of transitioning and discovering new parts of ourselves, as well as rediscovering ourselves and our interests. I asked my friend Catherine what it was like to have her youngest child leave the home, in hopes of preparing myself for when this time comes. Catherine said, "Signe, it's a little bit like death, you can prepare all you'd like but there's really no preparing for the weight of it once it happens. The only thing I can say is to nurture your life, figure out what it is you really want to do that makes you happy and brings you comfort that allows you to step away from the weight of it all. Honestly a lot of the things I've done to feather my nest are a little bit escapist, to just get away from the feeling."

SCENES FROM THE EMPTY NEST

by Catherine

There are moments our mothers never truly told us about, the experiences hidden in the shadows of our childhoods and carried with us as forbidden secrets carried quietly into adulthood. The way we knew we'd get a period; then experiencing the shock of flooding our underwear with bright red blood in big amounts everywhere – at school and at dances, or overnight at friends' houses. The way it felt to sink into the indulgent sensory overload of being in bed with a man. The jarring reality of having a baby, giving birth to two new humans – the child, and ourselves. And in our fatigue blending with the euphoria of baby love, sensing the pulse of all ancient mothers through time, cradling our child as they did, living with crying, feedings, and the rotating dizzying nights and days of this small, helpless, loud little being. The knowing of being mothers; and how it one day suddenly stops. One day there is loud chaos and a million details to remember and the next, it's quiet. There's a deep, aching void that our mothers never told us about, the quiet stillness of the house, when the last child leaves the home.

The nest now a fragmented pile of sticks where feathers and eggs once rested and chirping incessant beaks used to bob for food. Marriage itself, once obscured by so much dawn to dusk minutiae that it hardly warranted a moment's notice, now looming overhead like a big unwanted puzzle that asks to be completed, somehow. It's like a ripping of sorts; a focus cut short, a path suddenly ended by a felled tree.

The kids are gone.

Too much calling, writing, messaging, heck you could call it begging; and you drive them away. Too much drinking, overeating, pills or overwhelm and you will drive everyone away. So after the tears have dried, you sit with your head in your hands, and you drift. Backwards. Who were you before all this happened to you and life made you into a mother? Peel back the years. The memories are there. What did it feel like to live as a child? In preschool, you were three years old. What defined you as a person? What appealed to you? Did you dress up in clothes and pretend to be someone else? Did you spend hours gluing macaroni to paper? Did you delight in the dogs visiting or the horses in the field? What about books? What was it like to listen to music, and did the piano or the guitar call to you? Did you love shouting out songs? Making friends? Did you delight in fantasy and storytelling or did you love balancing and swinging from the bars in the playground?

Did your essential core self ever change? When we became mothers, it felt that way, for a long time. My motherhood lasted 27 years. From age 27 to 54. For 27 years all my focus, all my attention, all my love was poured into three people: My three daughters. Then suddenly, shockingly, it's over.

In 2021, my youngest child was still at home, but she was drifting from me. She didn't want my attention, my all-encompassing care. Meals I made languished in the refrigerator for days. I'd come home from work and she'd be out with friends or hidden away in her room. The hours drifted in the long afternoons that shifted into evenings. I mused about my childhood, remembering hours, weeks, months spent at the piano. I wondered, what would happen if I picked up a guitar every single day for a year? What if I learned to play all my favorite songs I loved to sing on the radio? Over that year, and three years later, I'd accumulated an electric guitar, an amp, two acoustics, and I'd learned to fingerpick melodies and use a pick to isolate notes. I wrote a song. I listened to my vocals and my brassy throaty tone became something softer, more even, more consistent. I played an open mic. I dreamed about more.

One year I used my own money from work to buy a van, which my husband converted into a camper. Over the last five years, I have driven off, driven away to immerse myself in nature. When the quiet, and the questions, and my work as a nurse threatened to swallow me whole, I would pack up the van and drive. Alone, with dogs. To the beach, the mountains, the desert. Then I drove one summer all the way to the east coast, staying in rest stops and truck stops along the way, driving through so many endless states for days on end it felt like my life was just a continuous drive. I motored through forests and deserts and plains, I drove through three time changes and heavy air with cicadas and masses of freeways and tolls, and lightning separating the dark skies with thunderstorms, until I'd reached my cousin's house in New York. Two summers later, I did it again.

I sit in this tattered nest with its broken twigs and smashed eggshells, a nest that once held so much life. I lay two or three soft, abundant feathers gently on top of those brittle branches. For a moment, I settle in, and these few feathers soften this moment of dark reverie. They are a cushion for the stark reality of this life that seems bereft of the surging, encompassing love that lived here, the millions of tiny yet not insignificant moments that filled up our lives, and the decades I spent as a mother.

Despite this incessant yearning for the past, this void that threatens to envelop me, this change thrust on me by none other than nature and the way of the world, there is no other real option for me. I'll find the child I forgot; the one I thrust aside in the name of adulthood and maturity, and let her loose in a field of flowers, laughing and careening around, with that loud voice that belts her music, shouting with glee as she picks up as many feathers as she can find.

What would happen if you gathered up all the love you used to give to your children – love that would smother them now, love bundled up like an armful of feathers – and gave all that love to yourself?

FEATHERING YOUR OWN NEST

If you find there are gaps in your friendship domain that you'd like to fill, where do you start? A client of mine said, "I know I need new friends, I can't exactly just go to 'the friend store.'" A good start is identifying the qualities you're looking for in a friendship. By midlife we know who we are and have years of experience regarding what works and doesn't work for us. In the book *The Science of Making Friends*, there are nine characteristics suggested when thinking about what entails a good friendship: The sharing of common interests, caring, support, mutual understanding, commitment and loyalty, honesty and trust, equality, ability to self-disclose, and the ability to resolve arguments and conflicts without hurting the friendship (conflict resolution) (Laugeson, 2013, pp. 38–42).

Next, take an inventory to get a feel for the types of friendship you're looking for. Are you looking for a friend to occasionally grab a movie with? A friend you can disclose your deepest thoughts and feelings to? What is the end in view for the friendship you are looking for? "Acquaintances are people we know slightly, casual friends are those we socialize with but aren't close to, regular friends are those that involve regular socializing and a slight degree of closeness, and close friends and best friends are those that involve frequent socializing and a high degree of closeness. These best friendships include most, if not all of the characteristics of good friendship" says Laugeson (Laugeson, 2013, p. 201).

In my interview with Laugeson she says, "Making new friends starts with you. What do you like to do? What are your interests? Who else likes to do these things? Where are they?" Social groups are essential to finding a potential source of friends, a way to feel connected to something larger than yourself" (Darpinian, 2022). She notes that we need to change our goals before going into a social setting; the goal shouldn't be to get along with everyone. We don't need to be friends with everyone, and not everyone needs to be friends with us. Just because we want to be friends with someone doesn't mean we get to and just because someone wants to be friends with us doesn't mean we have to (Laugeson, 2013, p. 37). Making your social goal more realistic when going into a group leads to less disappointment.

I learned about the idea of looking for "rainbows" in a social group from Intuitive Counselor, Holly Davies (Holly Marian Davies, 2025). Cheesy I know, but these are people that really see you and get you, and vice versa. Our rainbows are the people that bring out the best in us – and we bring out the best in them. It feels safe to be ourselves around these people. There are also bound to be "partial rainbows" in the group, people we have some commonalities with, such as similar work, and of course there will be some dark clouds. Ideally you be you, don't dim your light in the presence of dark clouds, and see if you can simply "gently avoid" them. Remember that friendship is a choice. Adopting this motto leads to healthier friendships overall.

Taking it personally when someone doesn't reciprocate wanting to be friends with us is very human since we are wired to belong, but do your best to use your emotions wisely and affirm, "I'm worthy of love and belonging whether this person wants to be my friend or not." Otherwise the brain will become overrun with stories we tell ourselves about not being enough for someone to want to stay. We all have these narratives, our "greatest hits," and they are often thought habits that are built on a faulty premise. Do your best to shift your gaze back to all of the rainbows you have in your life. Sometimes I write out every single rainbow, from the neighbors on my street, to the server at my local bakery, best friends and family members, just to remind myself how many there are.

EXPLORATION: FINDING YOUR RAINBOWS THROUGH MEETUP

Identifying the characteristics that are compatible with you, as well as the closeness you are looking for in a friendship, are essential starting places. The next step is rediscovering your interests and taking action toward seeing who else enjoys those things, too. Meetup is a global organization founded by Scott Heiferman in 2002. Back in 2001, Heiferman was living in downtown New York City. On September 11 of that year, he watched in horror along with millions of others as two planes crashed into the World Trade Center.

Prior to 9/11, Heiferman didn't have much of a relationship with his neighbors, but on that day he found comfort in their shared experience of grief and support. Those feelings inspired him to become more involved with his community in the aftermath, attending vigils and volunteering with the Red Cross at Ground Zero. In the wake of these events, and the profound sense of togetherness he discovered, Scott wondered how to continue authentically connecting people for good causes. His answer would be Meetup (Heieferman, 2024). Today, there are over 300,000 Meetup groups in more than 200 countries.

These groups revolve around a large array of interests from hiking, to technology, to book clubs.

Stevie came to therapy because her support system was lacking close and best friends. She was in postmenopause and no longer had kids at home, so finding and making new friends in this life stage was more difficult for her than it had been at any other stage of life. She lived in the San Francisco Bay Area, and loved to hike, so she found a Meetup hiking group that advertised, "Whether you're a seasoned hiker or just starting out, this group is for women who are interested in exploring the beauty of San Francisco Bay Area trails together!"

We did a "cope ahead" together so she could shift her mindset from wanting everyone in the group to like her, to a goal based more on the reality of making one or two close connections over time. She was committed to going to the Meetup twice a month and knew that it would take time to get familiar with the group.

Stevie felt her people skills were rusty so we practiced some skills together in session around the basics of entering a conversation, trading information, and exiting a conversation, another hallmark of the skills training at the UCLA PEERS clinic.

Here's a sample:

> *Stevie*: How long have you been coming to this group?
> *Meetup Attendee*: I've been coming for six months now.
> *Stevie*: Oh cool, this is my first time.
> *Meetup Attendee*: Do you live in the East Bay?
> *Stevie*: No, I actually live in San Francisco.
> *Meetup Attendee*: Oh wow, I grew up there...

You'll notice that looking for common interests in conversation naturally leads to trading information. This is a way to make friends with people you have things in common with. And of course, making new friends takes repetition, so Stevie will need to commit to attending the Meetup regularly until she becomes familiar with the other hikers. After some time with the group, Stevie might develop a closer connection with another hiker or two to have a get-together outside of the Meetup group.

EXPLORATION

What characteristics are important to you in a friend?
What kinds of friendships are you looking for?
What are your interests?
Where can you find other people that are interested in the same thing?

INTERGENERATIONAL FRIENDSHIPS

Pop culture has started to popularize intergenerational friendships (defined as having a 15-year age gap or more). Think of the dark mentorship-turned-friendship in the MAX show Hacks, between Las Vegas comic Deborah Vance (played by Jean Smart) and 25-year-old comedy writer Ava Daniels (played by Hannah Einbinder). "Friendship is a choice" doesn't mean we always make good choices. Or Rebecca Welton (played by Hannah Waddingham) and Keeley Jones (played by Juno Temple) in the Apple TV sports comedy Ted Lasso. When we first meet Keeley, she's a vivacious model-turned-publicist for football team AFC Richmond, and Rebecca, as the club owner, is her boss. Rebecca's character is in her mid-40s, and Keeley is a 30-year-old in the show. Rebecca teaches Keeley about the value of accountability in a romantic partner, wisdom she's imparting to Keeley after 12 years of her own marriage that lacked this value. Keeley teaches Rebecca how to find her confidence again as she's recovering from an abusive relationship. Keeley is exactly the breath of fresh air Rebecca needs to help her return to her true self. These two embody all the characteristics found in a healthy best friendship: The sharing of common interests in their work, genuinely caring for and supporting each other (having each other's backs), mutual understanding, and displays of treating each other with respect even when they might not like the other person's behavior – which illustrates one of the core characteristics at PEERs: The ability to resolve arguments and conflicts without hurting the friendship.

Intergenerational friendships at work in the real world offer knowledge, and it's often where intergenerational dialogues happen. The Menopause Society (TMS) has started a Making Menopause Work™ initiative. They say, "Midlife women are at the top of their game across jobs and sectors, are holders of institutional wisdom, mature in decision-making, and dynamic and influential leaders" (*Making Menopause Work*, 2025). Now that menopause is finally getting the attention it deserves, TMS is providing a template for companies to adopt a more "menopause responsive workplace." This can mean anything from being mindful of the temperatures at work to help with hot flashes, understanding brain fog, and making accommodations for heavy bleeding, to flexibility from a manager when a woman needs to leave work for an OB/GYN appointment.

TMS supports the idea that enhancing menopause literacy in the workplace means providing support for an important source of talent. Intergenerational friendships, personal or professional, are often a natural source of menopause information for younger women, and can provide anticipatory guidance around a topic that has historically been taboo to talk about. I'll never forget walks around the lake with my mentor, colleague, and friend Connie Sobczak, founder of The Body Positive. She would tell me about her menopause transition while I was still in my premenopause years. She normalized the body changes to come and talked to me about how she didn't necessarily feel invisible in midlife and beyond, though she said, "If I choose, and want to hide, I can hide more easily now." Said Sobczak, "If I think I'm not okay because I'm 61 years old, or because I'm aging, or I have gray hair – or whatever it is – then I'm going to be invisible. Bottom line is that I don't need to be seen by others in the same way I used to, because I see myself. And I like what I see!" (Darpinian, 2021)

I have a millennial friend who encourages me to take inspired action in life, and follow "what makes my soul sing." And a close Boomer friend who models maintaining family and friend-family relationships for me, and advises me about stages of life I've not lived yet, such as empty nesting and grandparenting. With up to three decades' more life experience and wisdom than I have, she can give me perspective to navigate difficult situations that seem dire at my life stage. These kinds of exchanges of perspectives and life experiences are the hallmark of cross-generational friendships.

REFERENCES

Darpinian, S. (2021, November 9). *The art of aging.* Therapy Rocks! https://audioboom.com/posts/7975329-the-art-of-aging

Darpinian, S. (2022, April 1). *The science of making friends.* Therapy Rocks! https://audioboom.com/posts/8055187-the-science-of-making-friends

Heieferman, S. (2024). Scott heiferman. In *Wikipedia.* https://en.wikipedia.org/w/index.php?title=Scott_Heiferman&oldid=1243561950

Holly Marian Davies. (2025). *Soulsageglobal.* SoulSageGlobal. https://soulsageglobal.com/holly-marian-davies

Laugeson, E. (2013). *The science of making friends: Helping socially challenged teens and young adults.* Wiley.

Making Menopause Work. (2025). The Menopause Society. https://menopause.org/workplace

Waldinger, R. (Director). (2015, November). *What makes a good life? Lessons from the longest study on happiness* [Video recording]. https://www.ted.com/talks/robert_waldinger_what_makes_a_good_life_lessons_from_the_longest_study_on_happiness

Nine

Healthy Romantic Relationships in Midlife and Beyond

Well, this is embarrassing. I conducted focus groups when I was prepping for my podcast interviews on menopause. I mapped out every theme and category I wanted to cover, and I felt like I knew what women would want to talk about. I was a Goddess of Preparation! At the end of one of the groups I casually asked, "Can you think of anything else you'd like me to bring up in my menopause interviews?" (Secretly thinking to myself, "How could they? I thought of everything!")

One woman hesitantly raised her hand and said, "Umm yes, what about sex?"

The others immediately chimed in with their agreement, and I realized I'd unwittingly overlooked a topic that does not lose its resonance or its relevance in midlife.

Sexual health (or sexual well-being) is important to our overall sense of self and well-being, whether we are in a partnership or single. There is no standard to meet when it comes to sexual activity and desire, which also means many of us are uncertain about our own sex lives. Are we "normal?" Having enough sex? More or less satisfied than our friends?

Research shows that some women experience a significant decline in sexual desire during midlife, and prefer to keep romance alive by seeking out novel experiences with their partner, and enjoying non-sexual intimacy such as hand holding. Others report an increased interest, and still others notice no change at all. Only you can know whether or not your sex life meets your needs. Every couple, and every individual, makes their own rules.

In my practice, it takes a strong therapeutic relationship before clients feel comfortable talking about their sexual health. This is

DOI: 10.4324/9781003632245-13

understandable. Therapist Dawn Serra says, "It's hard to talk about this thing we never 'see' except in the form of entertainment." Adds Serra, "The sex we see on TV or in films typically has a 'Las Vegasy' quality to it" (Darpinian, 2022). Participants are generally young and physically flawless (to our conditioned eye) and sex scenes are beautifully lit and balletically choreographed. Our media doesn't usually depict a robust sex life in midlife and beyond, although representation is slowly getting better (I'm looking at you Grace & Frankie).

If you're dealing with low sexual desire in menopause, know that you are not alone. Sexual health in midlife and beyond is multifactorial, meaning it's impacted by common social changes (caring for aging parents, changing partners, divorce, widowhood), body changes (low estrogen causes the vagina to become dry and less elastic), and fluctuating energy levels (night sweats can interrupt sleep, making sexual desire less of a priority). Many of the women I've worked with have received substantial help and support from therapists who specialize in treating sexual concerns. It might feel daunting, but these are professionals who talk about sex and sexuality every day. Don't be afraid to seek that support for yourself.

COMMON MIDLIFE RELATIONSHIP THEMES, HEALTHY LOVE, AND BEING SINGLE IN MIDLIFE AND BEYOND

by Dr. Brenda Schaeffer

According to Dr. Brenda Schaeffer, psychologist, and author of *Is It Love Or Is It Addiction?* midlife marks an important stage in our relationships, romantic or otherwise. Schaeffer notes, "At this stage of life couples in long term relationships experience transitions they have not planned for, such as empty nesting or going from busy lives to retirement. It's important to know what your vision is, and to share this vision with your partner. Do you plan to work until you're 75, while your partner wants to retire early and travel? In the business of life, many couples fail to talk about this. Or, they become so involved in other activities that they have stopped talking to each other and need to become reacquainted both with themselves and each other."

"Midlife is a prime time to reflect on old patterns and for those that don't work, to create new ones. It can be a time for growth. But the relationship has three entities: An 'I', a 'You', and a 'We'. The 'We' can only be as healthy as the 'I' and the 'You'. And that means it's time to stop doing other people's inventory and conduct our own. If you have not already done so, you need to examine yourself and ask such questions as, 'Why do I do or say the things I do?' 'Why am I such a people pleaser?' 'Why do I need to have control?' People can relax into their imperfections and, with humor, own that they do not have all of the answers to the life and love puzzle."

"We all have a bit of brokenness inside of us, and we unconsciously want our significant other to fix it. Our dysfunction has a source somewhere. None of us got everything we needed in just the way we needed it and that is a fact of life. We look to others to fill those unmet needs or heal our trauma, whatever it is. We unconsciously want others to fix the brokenness inside of us, and it's not their job. Even if they could fix us, if we have a core belief of 'I don't matter,' we won't take it in the good stuff given to us."

"When I witness those who have done the work to get to know themselves in midlife or before, they not only take responsibility for their dysfunctional behavior in the relationship, they begin to teach their partners about their emotional soft spots (sometimes called triggers.) They strive to be emotionally honest, and they are willing to share power."

"Here is an exercise to help in letting go of the old and embracing the new.

Honestly examine your role in the relationship.
Acknowledge resistance to change.
Stop looking for magic or external solutions to problems.
Look inward to examine fears, self promises, and archaic beliefs that support negative behaviors.
Reprogram negative beliefs and experiences.

If you need help with the above, make an agreement to find it. Therapy is a great way to get to know yourself and your partner better. You can learn to share and to communicate" (Darpinian, 2024).

WHAT IS HEALTHY LOVE?

We weren't exactly given a manual about what healthy love is. Most of our movies and media are based on the beginning or ending stages of a love relationship. A healthy love relationship isn't as sexy of a sell. Dr. Schaeffer summarizes:

> We know how to be attracted to someone and have chemistry, we know how to fall into romantic love, but, when all the chemicals wane, we aren't as good at the bonding stage of a relationship. Maybe our hearts have been hurt and we fear closeness. Maybe we have only a few pieces of a 100 piece relationship puzzle. Maybe our role models were ineffective. Love and relationships are not one and the same. Relationships are neutral places where we get to experience profound love as well as withhold it. Some relationships are toxic or mean. Some are addictive or highly dependent. Love is an energy that is free and available to all. It does not care if you are married, single, or in a relationship at all. But when love is in a relationship it nourishes; it is green and growing. The relationship moves beyond physical and romantic stages. It has a feeling of safety: safe to be me, safe to disagree, safe to have feelings and needs and safe to succeed. Safety generates a feeling of trust, which is the foundation of a healthy relationship. Congruence in word and action is an important aspect of trust. When one's thoughts and actions do not match, acknowledging the inconsistency can make them congruent. For example, "I love you but I have problems expressing love," puts a person into congruence.
>
> (Darpinian, 2024)

BODY POSITIVITY AS A RELATIONSHIP VALUE

You might be asking, "What does body positivity have to do with menopause?" Body positivity is often associated with conversations about body size. It's true: A big part of accepting your or someone else's body is accepting the parts of it that society judges. That might be the jiggliest parts, or the parts of us that have stretch marks. Body positivity doesn't stop there, though. Society judges menopause and the menopausal body, too. Body positivity is here to help you prioritize non-judgment and acceptance as your body changes. Body positivity is a value that you can adopt for yourself, and it's also a value that you can bring into and expect from your friendships and relationships.

Virgie is in a self-proclaimed "body positive marriage," which she has valued as a plus-size, fat-positive feminist. One of her long-time mantras has been "trust your body," but when she began having intense, prolonged perimenopausal bleeding in her early forties, she began to question whether there were exceptions to her rule. She also found herself wondering whether her spouse's body positive values had room for bloody sheets. In the next section she shares her story.

NO ONE TOLD ME ABOUT THE BLOODBATH

by Virgie Tovar

This story starts with blood on sheets.

At 41 years old, I – a plus-size, fat-positive, anti-diet, Mexican-Iranian with chubby cheeks, blunt cut bangs, a great big laugh, and pink oversized wayfarer glasses – started having bloody blowouts. Blood would just gush out in such volume and so quickly that a pad (even one of those humongous overnight ones) simply wasn't designed to keep up. This would happen on places like the sofa, while I was watching TV. Just: Gush, and there it was, an enormous bloody stain on a huge patch of fabric. Then came the sheets: Soaked and in need of changing day after day after day.

I share my bed (and my sheets) with my husband, Andrew. I met Andrew in my mid-thirties. By then, I had come full circle in my relationship with my body. I had gone from hating my fat body and trying desperately to lose weight by any means necessary, which led to an eating disorder in my early twenties to deciding, in my late twenties and early thirties, that I wanted to celebrate my body, never diet again, and, while I was at it, try to end weight-based discrimination in the culture.

I was also over a decade into my body positive dating practice. For me, this primarily consisted of a Zero Fatphobia Tolerance dating policy. The policy worked like this: No matter how long I'd been dating someone, if they said anything negative about my body size or how I ate, I would dump them. I highly recommend this policy! It certainly changed my life for the better.

Andrew has a lot of magical qualities, but my favorite one is that some part of him was just never truly destroyed by misogyny or crushing societal norms. He doesn't see people through the lens of hierarchy or personal gain. He doesn't see women as glorified servants or trophies. He just sees people. And he sees me as the rotund, cute, and mischievous creature I am, not what society renders me as: Ugly, fat, and loud.

Yes, like me, Andrew is fat positive or body positive.

Typically – though not always – body positivity is a value that clusters with other values and traits that I think make for a good relationship. In general, I've found people who want to be in serious, egalitarian relationships with fat people (or other marginalized groups) are more comfortable with non-conformity and are less incentivized by cultural approval.

Back to blood.

Now, I'm not one to really hide her period. As a feminist and a generally oversharey person, I don't believe in discretely tucking my pad away when I'm in public, nor do I think my husband should be "spared" the sight of blood if he walks into the bathroom to brush his teeth while I'm peeing and my pad is out for the whole world to see. We have sex while I'm on my period as well.

He has a proven track record of loving (nay, worshiping) my fat body, but I have to admit I never really thought about whether all this menses was pushing his body positive stance, or even if his body positive outlook included menopause. Frankly, I hadn't thought much of menopause at all. When I did think of it, I imagined it as a creek unceremoniously going dry one day. I'd never even heard of perimenopause before I was knee-deep in uterine lining. My grandma used to talk to me about the emotional side of menopause for her and how sad she was that she was no longer reproductive. As someone who never much liked the idea of reproduction, it seemed like a one-way ticket out of nuisance-ville. Nary was there a word about the bloodbath!

I bled for days, then weeks, then months. I was more annoyed than alarmed. I dogmatically believed in trusting my body come hell or high water. So, I rationalized that any day now, my body, in its infinite wisdom, would stop on its own. I never felt light-headed or anything, but my relationship to food started to get really weird. I was eating all the time. I love eating and I do not believe there is a "right" way to eat, but I could tell something was off for me. I felt compelled to eat in a way that was totally disconnected from hunger, fullness, or desire. It was around this time that I went on a short trip with a friend, and we shared a room. I mentioned that there may be blood everywhere, but not to be alarmed.

"Wait, how long have you been bleeding?" she asked.

"Oh, I don't know, maybe two or three months," I replied, trying to downplay how bad I knew that sounded.

Her eyebrows shot up. "No, no, no, girl. You need to have this looked at immediately." We discovered we were in the same network of medical care providers. She promptly gave me the name of her OB/GYN and made sure to watch as I initiated a new patient request.

During my appointment, my new OB/GYN ordered some bloodwork, put me on birth control (reminder that you can still get pregnant in perimenopause) and a daily regimen of 50 mg of iron per day. It took a few weeks, but the bleeding stopped. My bloodwork showed that I was anemic. It wasn't long after I started taking iron that my relationship with food went back to my normal. I realized the reason that my eating had gotten weird was because my smart body was trying to get the iron I was losing vaginally, from food. I felt so grateful for all the work my body had done to keep me both alive and upright.

Nowadays, my periods are much less intense and my body is no longer desperately trying to pull iron from food. Oh, and I got a really big, fat, thick blanket, which I fold in two and sleep on (on my side of the bed) if I have a particularly heavy flow for a day or two. It's just my bloody blanket now. No more bloody sheets.

When it comes to whether my bloodbath pushed the limits of Andrew's body positivity, maybe it did. But never did I get a single wrinkled nose, raised eyebrow or refusal to have sex. Never did he suggest I needed a new menstrual management system. Never once did he say a judgmental word.

"Bodies are gross" is something Andrew says often, lovingly, and with a little smile. This might not sound very "positive," but accepting the gross bits is the hard part. Those are the bits that require our acceptance. Sometimes body positivity seems like a lofty, tidy or heady ideal, but really it's just the acceptance of life: Hair, sweat, zits, and shits. Oh, and blood. Lots of blood.

SINGLE IN MIDLIFE

In my interview with Dr. Schaeffer, I asked how a person might know if they are single for the right or wrong reasons. She said, "It's important to know the difference. Being single for the right reason is a choice. Perhaps a person wants more time to examine themself and the choices they make. Or, a romantic relationship has ended via death or divorce, and a person wants time to grieve. Or a person genuinely enjoys their singleness and the positives it brings: More time for self-care, career, friendships, family, or other pursuits. Someone who is single for the right reasons might say, 'I am comfortable with myself and my life. If the right person comes along, I am game. I am happy with or without a partner.'"

Schaeffer says, "Being single for the wrong reason is based on fear. A person is love avoidant because they were hurt, abandoned, betrayed, minimized, rejected, or abused, and fear a repeat. Or, a person does not trust that they will take good care of themselves in a relationship. Or they distrust their ability to make good choices. Some relationships may have been so traumatic that they fear they may not be able to trust again. The anti-dependent stance may involve fewer risks of being hurt or disappointed, but it can also feel lonely. Being single for the right or wrong reason is an opportune time to dig into our history or personal life script, heal old wounds, and examine outdated beliefs and behaviors. It's soul searching time. Early experiences determine who we love and what we believe about love. We learn more about what love is not than what love is: love is hurt, love is betrayal, love is earned, love is not there for me. Unless we find and rewire these beliefs, we are likely to unconsciously find relationships that support such beliefs."

"Let's face it. Any time we are in a relationship we are vulnerable. We need to be strong enough and love ourselves enough to take risks and ask for what we need without expectations. You might get the answer you want and you might not. But celebrate that you asked. The more we understand our behavior, the more we have control over it.

The lessons we learn help us to develop emotional maturity, self-trust, self-esteem, which leads to healthier love relationships."

EXPLORATION: WHAT LESSONS HAVE YOU LEARNED IN LOVE?

Eg. I notice that when someone makes me feel too needy, I tend to take it personally instead of acknowledging that it's a sign of an emotionally unavailable person. In the future, if someone makes me feel too needy, I will notice it at the first sign and move on (Darpinian, 2024).

MAKE A LIST!

We don't begin our lives knowing exactly what we are looking for in a partner. We arrive at realizations about what works for us and what doesn't via experience – much in the same way we've learned to listen to our boundaries and honor them, instead of waiting for them to take care of themselves. An advantage of dating in midlife is that we have had many opportunities to gain the wisdom we need to recognize old relationship patterns, acknowledge them, and walk away.

If you find yourself single in midlife and beyond, and feel happy with or without a relationship, but would like one, make a list! Stay focused on attributes you know you're looking for in a partner. When a potential candidate comes forward, go through a preliminary sorting process by checking out what you know about them as compared to your list. If there is more on the list that matches than not, and it feels right, move forward.

The list needs to stay current, so if you learn a lesson about something that does or does not work for you, add it to the list. Revisit the list regularly; it will help you stay focused on what you've learned. When I work with women in therapy on their list, I find it to be a helpful intervention when they are not in the first stages of getting to know someone. When chemistry is heightened we tend to ignore red flags.

Mantra: "The person I am ready to have a relationship with will show up easily and effortlessly and I'm ready for them now. I ask that our schedules blend and our paths cross in divine timing."

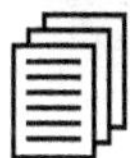

Sample Partner List

1. A person who values body positivity/size diversity
2. Has a diet-free lifestyle
3. Speaks straight, is not afraid to have difficult conversations
4. Someone who wants a serious relationship
5. Someone who is responsive, gets back to me in timely manner
6. Social drinking only
7. Willing to seek outside help if needed
8. Age range: 55–60
9. Has compatible values
10. Geographically desirable

If you ignore your list and decide to enter into a revolving door, ask yourself, "What is so enticing that I'm ignoring what I know to be my truth as it relates to someone I'd like to be with?" (Holly Marian Davies, 2025)

Partner List

1.

2.

3.

4.

5.

6.

7.

8.

9.

10.

DATING IN MIDLIFE WIDOWHOOD

by Dr. Linda Shanti

I remember making my first outreach call for grief support after my husband died. I had just turned 47 and was calling to inquire about joining a "Young Widows' Group." I didn't know if I fit the criteria, but I did know that the other widows' group had women in their 70s, 80s, and 90s. They were retired, they weren't currently raising children, and they weren't interested in talking about dating (or sex! or remarrying! Or choosing to be in a relationship and not get married!). The young widows' group, however, even had women in their twenties (yes, there are women that are widowed in their twenties).

I thought, "Am I in no-man's land?" I spoke with the young widows' group facilitator and asked, "Am I going to be the oldest in the room? Do I still qualify?"

She was a kind, wise, and humorous woman who had been widowed in her thirties and was now in her sixties. She laughingly reassured me, "No, actually, I probably will be!" She welcomed me into the group, and there were other middle aged widows also wrestling with challenges around parenting, perimenopause, careers, and dating.

Dating, for those midlife widows who choose to, is often a very different experience than the experience we had dating our late spouse. Many of us last dated when we were much younger, often before the rise of "the apps." We had met our spouse in real life, gotten to know them, and built a life together. Our life goals at that time were likely very different and included such goals as finishing our education, starting our career, buying a house, and having children. Midlife women are in a very different stage. We are often more solid in our careers, have already had our children, and know with more certainty who we are, and who we are not. We may have more financial freedom and more clarity in what does and does not interest us. In addition, even though we may know ourselves better, many of us are also asking the question "Who am I, now, without my person?" which takes time and effort to discover.

Compare and Despair

One of the most common experiences for widows who choose to date is to compare their dates with their spouse who died. I don't think it's a problem to compare, but it is a problem to *despair about* the comparison. Here is the thing: You will never meet your late spouse again, and you will probably always feel sad about that...*and* (that is the magic word) you can also love another person just as much, in a different way (because they are a different person). In addition, YOU are not the same person as you were when you met your late spouse, so YOU are different! Yes, you might be more cynical and feel broken. And you are also more brave, experienced, more of a badas*, and yes, more broken – more broken open. One might say your heart is even bigger because of it. Here are a few more thoughts about dating as a midlife widow.

Getting Over It Versus Going On

Many people believe that the best way to "get over" your late spouse is to "move on" from grief, date, and "replace" them. But people aren't replaceable. When you say "you should get over it and move on" to a widowed person, what they often hear is:

"There is something wrong with you if you feel sad that your person died. That makes me uncomfortable. Please forget your person, get over it, date someone else, and move on, so I don't feel uncomfortable."

We don't move on from grief. And grief is uncomfortable: For the griever and for the grief adjacent. You can, however, bring the love and memories you have for your person with you, as you move forward, sharing love and making memories with another person.

Other People's Opinions

Nowhere are other people's opinions of widows more apparent than judgments about "what is right/not right" about dating – usually coming from people who have not walked the path of widowhood. Some people think (fill in their opinion on length) is the right time, some people think (fill in opinion on length) is too soon, some people think (fill in opinion on length) is too long to wait. For widows, your dating experience, and your dating timeline, like your grief experience, is *your individual experience*. Only you know when the right time to date is, for you. Feel free to leave the opinions of other people out of your decision-making process.

You're Not Cheating on Them

Most people don't think about the "'til death do us part" part of their marriage vows until it happens. And then, if you were happily married, it can feel surreal to be dating...or kissing...or having sex with another person who is not your spouse. It can feel like you are cheating on them.

You're not. You fulfilled your vows. You get to decide what to do, who to be with, and in what way, from here. It's okay if that feels strange, great, awful, or some combination of all those things. (Also, some widows experience "widow's fire," a phenomenon in which their libido is very high, often during acute grief. If you have this experience, it doesn't mean you're a slut, unfaithful or abnormal.)

What if You Like Them, and They Die, Too?

Even though it is 100 percent guaranteed that everyone you love (and you) will die, death is not something for which our culture prepares us. And so, when it happens to our loved one, we are left shocked and reeling. The death of our loved one, and the lifelong process of grief, shatters what psychologists call our "assumptive world." When your person dies, it can shatter your foundation of trust and safety in the world and cause you to wonder if you want to risk that kind of love again. This is a very big risk. (For what it's worth, in my opinion, it's worth it.)

Happy, Even After

I remember getting into my car after I went on my very first coffee date after my husband died. I swore and cried. I felt so very shocked and sad. I did not like this date, and it felt so weird to be sitting across from someone at Starbucks, on a first date, at age 48. I have been on many coffee dates since then, some fabulous, some meh. I have met some very interesting people! None of them (so far) are my next person. I mention this because two other myths are: You will meet the next person you marry on your first date, and you can only write inspirational dating stories after you have successfully found and married your next person. Like the "it's complicated" status on Facebook, most people, widowed or not, have a lifetime of experiences – aka baggage – that they bring with them when dating in middle age. I don't believe it is helpful to try and get rid of this baggage or make it small enough to fit in the overhead compartment. I think it is more about knowing what is inside your baggage. Once you know that, you can release the shame about the parts you don't like and love the heck out of the gifts you have to offer.

For those of us who have experienced the death of our person, and grieved deeply, it means we have the capacity to love deeply. If you choose to date again, it is not a matter of your baggage making you broken, or there not being someone that is a good fit for you. It is a matter of you becoming the person you want to be, and then finding the right person with whom to share that big, broken-open love. Sometimes that is with someone else, sometimes that is with YOU. Either way (or both), I do know, because I've experienced it, that it's totally possible to be happy, even after.

Not everyone grieving needs to go to a grief support group. Not everyone who loses their person needs to go to a professional for grief counseling. We want to be mindful not to pathologize grief; it is a universal experience. And even though it is universal, the way people experience it is individual.

David Kessler says, "People grieve in character." So if someone is introverted, they may not feel comfortable in a support group setting, and individual grief counseling might be preferred, if needed. Those lacking a support system might choose to seek professional support. The instances that grief therapy and/or professional support would be recommended are: If your person died in a traumatic way and you're experiencing symptoms interfering in daily functioning, as a result of that trauma, and if you find grief is still impairing your quality of life one year after your person died.

REFERENCES

Darpinian, S. (2022, August 1). *Let's talk about sex...* Therapy Rocks! https://audioboom.com/posts/8130249-let-s-talk-about-sex

Darpinian, S. (2024, April 8). *Healthy relationships in midlife & beyond*. Therapy Rocks! https://audioboom.com/posts/8487626-healthy-relationships-in-midlife-beyond

Holly Marian Davies. (2025). *Soulsageglobal*. SoulSageGlobal. https://soulsageglobal.com/holly-marian-davies

Conclusion

New Age

Once I slapped on the estrogen patch and initiated nightly oral progesterone, my outlook on life, relationships, and the world shifted. It brightened. Clouds labeled anxiety, joint pain, and hot flashes drifted apart to reveal the golden, shining sun that had always been there, simply obscured. I could now keep my turbulent "greatest hits" at bay, having more access to my Wise Mind.

My relationship with my teenager shed its thin layer of vulnerability and returned to the baseline we had always securely enjoyed, now even better! (She no longer had to be my emotional support animal slash tea-bringer.) I brought new empathy and clarity to sessions with my clients, and new insights to my speaking engagements. I was able to play tennis without joint pain and can proudly report that I am a wonderfully…*average* athlete. When I wearied of waiting for the results from a messy hair restoration treatment, I decided instead to wear a short version of my wanna-be rocker 'do, and I made my way to the "indifference" end of Luciana's hair spectrum.

Life carried on. Life improved by the day. Life was once again a challenge and a blessing and a genuine delight. And once I felt this way, I wanted to make sure as many other women as possible could also flourish in this phase of life.

A great gift of my professional life has been the opportunity to deep dive into topics that interest me – in this case a topic I'm experiencing personally – and become closely acquainted with the research, the nuances, the personal stories, and the hopeful opportunities. Hosting my podcast and publishing my previous books *No Weigh! A Teen's Guide to Positive Body Image, Food, and Emotional Wisdom* and *Raising Body Positive Teens: A Parent's Guide to Diet-Free Living, Exercise and Body Image* have been

DOI: 10.4324/9781003632245-14

intellectually stimulating and allowed me to explore themes that mean the most to me.

Writing *A Woman's Guide to Menopause, Body Image, and Emotional Well-Being in Midlife* has taught me so much, and in turn I am hopeful that it can serve many different purposes for many different readers. Hewing to my professional background and closely held values, I wanted to explore midlife through a weight-inclusive lens, pushing back against the most harmful stereotypes and internet snake oil, in favor of practical, evidence-based strategies for physical and emotional wellness. I have addressed "protective factors" for risk factors related to disordered eating and body image dissatisfaction in midlife. If these strategies don't specifically apply to your life, chances are you know someone they might assist.

At the outset of my research and writing, my goal was to curate a toolbox for midlife and beyond, to help us all collectively reach a place of life satisfaction and presence, and especially to enjoy the accumulated wisdom that comes with midlife. I bring a gentle authority to this book, as a professional psychotherapist as well as someone with lived experience. I endeavored to walk alongside readers through the fundamentals of the menopause transition and provide valuable coping tools for the most common mood related symptoms – those that tend to upend our lives and require the most TLC. Midlife can be a confusing and isolating era, but it does not have to be. The community of shared experience starts within these pages.

If I could hand you this book's key takeaways on a silver platter, they would be:

Menopause and midlife can come with their own physical symptoms to address, and finding the right care and prioritizing oneself is key. There is no need to suffer in silence!

Emotional health in midlife and beyond is equally important, and myriad strategies exist to set us up for positive mental health and self-support.

Challenges and experiences around food and body image are as prevalent as ever in this era. The more things change, the more they stay the same, but the last thing we need in midlife is more diet culture. I've explored ways we can love ourselves and be loved for ourselves, live weight-inclusive lives, move our bodies joyfully, and intuitively eat the things that we love, which nourish us physically and emotionally.

Finally, and most crucially: This era of our lives is different but there is beauty in the differences – in sex, in friendship, in our bodies, in emotions, and even in love. I invite you to hone in on yourself and listen intuitively so that you can "come back home to yourself." Ask for help when you need it; you are worthy of love and support. Celebrate sustaining relationships or seek fulfilling new ones, and nurture your powerful rainbow friendships. Revel in the wisdom and knowledge that comes with midlife and beyond.

Coda

The Birth of My Feminine Self

Written by Victoria

As I sit here in my favorite spot, taking in the natural beauty of the Bay, I reflect upon my life's journey and the pathways that were set before me by divine intervention. The stepping-stones that guided me to the reality that is my life today. It is of no wonder to me today that I would be successful in my quest for a full and satisfying life, as my mother, who raised us, was and still is at age 91, a phenomenal woman. It is, however, thought-provoking how my socialization from early childhood, educational achievements, and physical health have shaped the resilient woman I have become.

I was once asked in a workplace meeting as an icebreaker, if you could have lunch with anyone in the world, who would it be? Without hesitation I responded, "My mother." Even though single parent households are commonplace in the 21st century, only eight percent of families were headed by a single parent at the time of my parents' divorce. The courage, tenaciousness, intellectual fortitude, and physical might required of this petite southern Black woman to raise and provide college educations for four children, while achieving her own doctoral degree, is nothing short of extraordinary. It would be an affront if I failed to point out that she worked full time and managed our home top to bottom…no nannies, no housekeepers. She persevered despite the stigma of divorce, and the institutionalized racism and misogyny within the educational institutions where she studied, taught, and ultimately retired as a college dean.

National and local accolades acknowledging her work in organizational leadership spanning her career hang on the walls of her home office, artifacts from her world travels adorn her home and shelf after shelf of literary works create a library rich in knowledge. Regardless of her undeniable exceptionalism, we witnessed how she was treated with disrespect and overlooked for promotions in the workplace. We wondered why store personnel seemed to be wherever we were when we shopped in upscale department stores. The life lessons learned from these observed prejudices, and the management of those inequities, served me well as I entered adulthood.

While I was able to engineer a successful career for myself, my ascension into leadership positions came with some of the same obvious and painful disparities. My educational accomplishments and experience often exceeded those of my colleagues; I wasn't afforded the opportunity of work-life balance when others were. I faced stereotypes of a pervasive caste system both in the workplace and our communities. I was expected to always have a smile on my face because I "looked angry." This was based on nothing tangible, it was simply how others felt! The weaponization of the "Angry Black Woman" stereotype is still widely employed to demean and create a false narrative of unworthiness.

My dark brown skin, full lips, and ample derrière rendered me unattractive and therefore undesirable based on the social constructs of the world I grew up in. I was not supposed to be successful let alone be loved, but I persisted, determined to fulfill my dreams; a career woman, wife, and mother. Someone gave me a gift many years ago, it was a framed quote that said, "She believed she could, so she did." It became my mantra. I believed if I persevered, I could achieve any goal that I had set and envisioned for myself. I established and grew my career in healthcare by 24 years of age. And so when I met and married my former spouse in my mid-30s I was ecstatic. I was on the threshold of having the full and well-rounded life I had imagined.

But it wasn't to be. I hadn't noticed that my body was changing. I hadn't noticed that I was becoming irritable and not sleeping through the night. I did however notice that my hair was thinning, and I was starting to put on a few pounds but nothing significant. Suddenly, at 35 years old, my menstrual cycle ceased to be, and I was diagnosed with premature ovarian failure (a disorder now medically described as primary ovarian insufficiency). I was devastated, but again I pushed forward. Given my background in healthcare, I knew that we had options and the decision to conceive through in vitro fertilization was a viable alternative for us. The months turned into years. Hormone injections and failed pregnancies reduced me to an emotional and physical wreckage. My body had been strained to its physical limits, I developed an endocrine disorder, hypertension, and became prediabetic. My marriage fell apart and there I was again, that little girl feeling unloved and undesirable, but this time I was a failure as well.

Months of therapy and years working with my healthcare team to address my newfound diagnoses left me feeling vulnerable, and generally skeptical about life. How would I manage my expectations going forward? I can't say that I had any at that point. It was all I could do to maintain the status quo at work and continue to be a good steward of my finances. I had learned that nothing was guaranteed, and that life was a bumpy road full of uncertainties.

The next five plus years were spent regaining my sense of self-worth and focusing on my health. I immersed myself in work, so dating was the furthest thing from my mind. But as life would have it, someone very special crossed my path; his name was Kai. I had moved and he was my neighbor who lived across the very small courtyard. He was 20 years my junior, so I never considered him to be a love interest. We struck up a conversation one random day a year later, and quickly became good friends over the next two years, chatting almost daily. The third year was the turning point for our emerging relationship. Unlikely as it might have been, we were soul mates, sharing all that we had to give. Life was exciting and fun; he was my person. Like myself, Kai was an ambivert; he enjoyed hanging out with close friends and family, but relished the serenity of home. We spent the next three years creating memorable experiences, and loving one another.

Kai passed away unexpectedly, and as horrific as his untimely death was, it was amplified by his proposal of marriage that had come just four months earlier. How would I even begin to process the magnitude of such a loss? I had no answers, but one thing was crystal clear, this was no time to be "superwoman," I needed help. I spent the next year (Mondays at 2!) learning how to grieve Kai's loss in a manner that was healthy, seeking to understand the whys, leaning into self-awareness and arriving at a place of peace. And while his death was heartbreaking, he left me with the most precious of gifts, he encouraged me to embrace my femininity.

Kai loved my smooth dark chocolate skin, full lips, and natural curves. He believed women should be soft and wholesome. I often found him watching me with his signature smile as I moved about the house. He always said that there was power in my femininity; I would look at him quizzically not quite believing him. One afternoon while out watching a basketball championship game in a hotel lounge, Kai chose that moment to show me that I garnered plenty of attention by simply being me. I had worn a modest sleeveless black top, with black slacks and sandals – I'm a firm believer that less is more. He leaned in close and whispered in my ear, "Walk over to the bar, order a couple of cocktails, and then just wait." Out of the periphery of my vision, I observed the gazes turned to stares around the room, who's that they eyed with curiosity? I giggled to myself and thought, hmmm, Kai's point was well taken. That was the beginning of my metamorphosis, stepping into and owning my femininity in the face of all my imperfections.

Do I still have thinning hair where it was once plentiful, nights of clammy insomnia, and the seemingly unreasonable bouts of irritability on occasion – absolutely! But I found that rejoicing in self-love and acceptance is a powerful thing. I no longer feel constrained by contrived attitudes based on intolerance. I'm unwavering when advocating for myself and able to constructively process whatever new changes my body may challenge me with. And my natural features, that once declared me as undesirable...yep, the very ones that brought about so much humiliation are now highly coveted. I take delight in my uniqueness and no longer crave the validation of arbitrary societal characterizations.

You may ask whether or not my life is the full and well-rounded life I envisioned for myself decades ago. I would say that I have been blessed beyond measure. My life has been robust with the love of five godchildren, graced by the riches of healthy relationships, and strengthened by a legacy of spirited women and evolved mentors. I celebrate the smart, emotionally intelligent, and courageous woman I have become...the culmination of personal evolution, tenacity, and grace. The good news, I'm not done yet! There are far more moments when I walk a little taller, chin up and shoulders back knowing that I am worthy of love and leaning into my reality.

In Loving Memory

Further Reading on Menopause

THE MENOPAUSE SOCIETIES

International Menopause Society: https://www.imsociety.org
The Menopause Society: https://menopause.org
Finding a Menopause Practitioner: https://portal.menopause.org/NAMS/NAMS/Directory/Menopause-Practitioner.aspx

BIPOC MENOPAUSE RESOURCE

Black and Menopausal: https://us.jkp.com/products/black-and-menopausal

TRANSGENDER AND GENDER DIVERSE HEALTH CARE AND MENOPAUSE RESOURCES

UCSF Transgender Care: Website: https://transcare.ucsf.edu/
Menopause in Gender Diverse Individuals: https://www.versalie.com/blogs/learn/menopause-gender-diverse-people
LGBTQ+ Healthcare Directory: https://lgbtqhealthcaredirectory.org/
Outlist LGBTQ+ Affirming Healthcare Directory: https://www.outcarehealth.org/outlist/
World Professional Association for Transgender Health (WPATH) Provider Directory: https://app.wpath.org/provider/search
Rock My Menopause: https://rockmymenopause.com/get-informed/transgender-health/
Queer Menopause: https://www.queermenopause.com/resources

WIDOWHOOD IN MIDLIFE

Dr. Linda Shanti, author of *After Your Person Dies*. Website: https://www.drlindashanti.com

WEIGHT-INCLUSIVE MIDLIFE NUTRITION

Val Schonberg, RD, MSCP, CSSD, website: https://valschonberg.com/

Jenn Salib Huber, RD, ND, CIEC author of *Eat To Thrive During Menopause: Managing Your Symptoms with Nourishing Foods*. Website: https://www.jennsalibhuber.ca/

Julie Dillon Duffy MS, RD, NCC, CEDS-C, author of *Find Your Food Voice: Defy Diet Culture, Declare Body Liberation, and Reclaim Your Peace*. Website: https://julieduffydillon.com/about/

Deb Benfield, M.Ed., RDN/LDN, RYT, author of *Unapologetic Aging: How to Mend and Nourish Your Relationship with Your Body*. Website: https://www.debrabenfield.com/about

Wendy Sterling, MS, RD, CSSD, CEDS-C, author of *How to Nourish Yourself Through an Eating Disorder: Recovery for Adults with the Plate-by-Plate Approach®*. Website: https://sterlingnutrition.com

Fiona Sutherland, Accredited Practising Dietitian (APD), RYT, The Mindful Dietitian. Website: https://www.themindfuldietitian.com.au

WEIGHT-INCLUSIVE MIDLIFE MEDICAL CARE

Weight Inclusive Menopause Practice: Seattle Menopause Medicine, website: https://www.seattlemenopause.com/

Lesley Williams, MD, MSCP: Eating disorder and menopause specialist who provides weight-inclusive trainings to clinicians wanting to implement these principles into their menopause practice: www.lesleywilliamsmd.com

Gaudiani Clinic, founded by Dr. Jennifer Gaudiani, author of *Sick Enough: A Guide to the Medical Complications of Eating Disorders and Undernourishment* (2nd Ed). Website: https://www.gaudianiclinic.com

Medical Students for Size Inclusivity (MSSI): https://sizeinclusivemedicine.org/

SLEEP RESOURCES

Ashley Brauer, Licensed Clinical and Sport Psychologist (PhD), and Diplomate in Behavioral Sleep Medicine (DBSM): https://drashleybrauer.com/

Cognitive Behavioral Therapy Insomnia (CBT-I) International Directory: https://cbti.directory/

PODCASTS

Therapy Rocks! a personal growth podcast
https://audioboom.com/channels/5020027-therapy-rocks
Hosted by Signe Darpinian, LMFT, CEDS

OvaryActive - A Podcast about Perimenopause
Co-hosts Amy J Voedisch, MD, MS, MSCP, and Rebecca Dunsmoor-Su, MD, MSCP

The Midlife Feast podcast
https://www.menopausenutritionist.ca/podcast
Hosted by Dr. Jenn Salib Huber RD, ND, CIEC

PELVIC FLOOR PHYSICAL THERAPY

Dr. Anietie Ukpe-Wallace, PT, DBT, author of *Tending to Your Womb: A Journey of Joy, Grief and Self-Discovery.* Website: https://www.selfcarephysio.com/

Pelvic Floor Physical Therapist (PFPT) of Color Directory: https://www.vaginarehabdoctor.com/woc-pfpt-directory/

Index

For Product Safety Concerns and Information please contact our EU representative GPSR@taylorandfrancis.com
Taylor & Francis Verlag GmbH, Kaufingerstraße 24, 80331 München, Germany

www.ingramcontent.com/pod-product-compliance
Lightning Source LLC
Chambersburg PA
CBHW071742270326
41928CB00013B/2771

* 9 7 8 1 0 4 1 0 5 3 1 8 7 *